First Printing, 2020.
ISBN 13: 978-1-84481-033-8
ISBN 10: 1-84481-033-X

Warning and Disclaimer
Although every precaution has been taken to verify the accuracy of the information contained herein, the author and publisher assume no responsibility for any errors or omissions. No liability is assumed for damage or injury that may result from the use of information contained within.

Fitness is a journey, not a destination.
Darebee Project

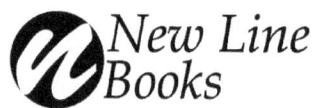

New Line
Books

New Line Books, London

Author Bio

Neila Rey is the founder of Darebee, a global fitness resource. She is committed to democratizing fitness by removing the barriers to it and increasing accessibility. Every workout published in her books utilizes the latest in exercise science and has undergone thorough field testing and refinement through Darebee volunteers. When she's not busy running Darebee she is focused on finding fresh ways to make exercise easier and more enjoyable.

1. Cardio

Get your blood pumping and your heart racing with this fast cardio routine on day one.

The better your form, the harder it gets. High Knees should be performed with the knees coming up to your waist each time (remember to land on the ball of the foot each time your foot comes down). When doing burpees try and go as high up in the air as you can.

Athena's PLAYBOOK

© darebee.com

Day 1 | Cardio

Level I 3 sets
Level II 5 sets
Level III 7 sets

2 minutes rest between sets

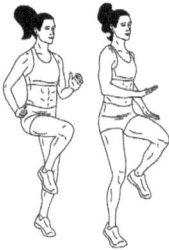

20 high knees

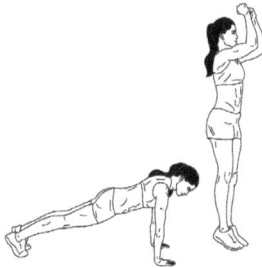

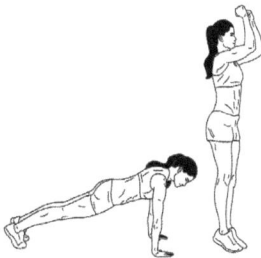

4 basic burpees

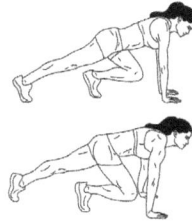

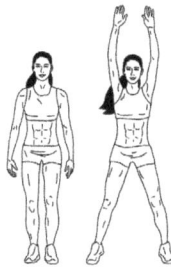

20 climbers

4 basic burpees

20 jumping jacks

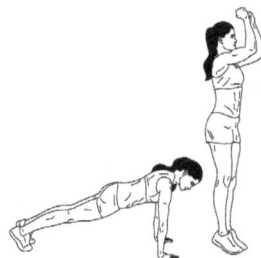

4 basic burpees

2. Upper Body

Upper body strength and power takes a lot of work. Focus on your moves, feel how your body moves in each exercise. Muscle awareness leads to better form and better results, faster.

Drive your punches with your core and feet. Push off the floor with the foot on the same side as the arm you're punching with. Twist your upper body in harmony with the push to generate power in your punch. Exhale lightly with each punch.

Athena's PLAYBOOK

© darebee.com

Day 2 | Upper Body

Level I   3 sets
Level II 5 sets
Level III 7 sets

2 minutes rest between sets

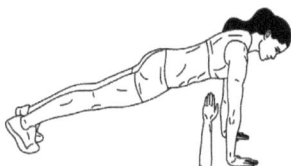

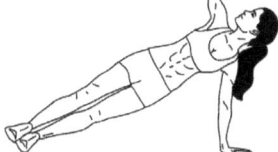

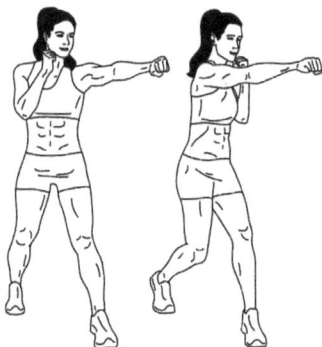

4 plank rotations

20 punches

4 plank rotations

20 punches

4 plank rotations

20 punches

4 plank rotations

20 punches

done

3. Lower Body

A strong lower body makes everything easier. It resists fatigue, generates more power and delivers speed when you need it the most.

Lower body strength springs from muscles, tendons and ligaments and the exercises on day three target them all.

Athena's PLAYBOOK

© darebee.com

Day 3
Lower Body

2 minutes rest
between exercises

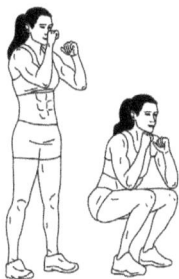

10 squats **x 3 sets** in total
20 seconds rest between sets

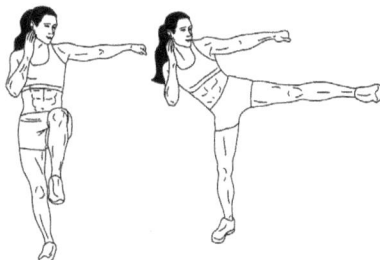

20 side kicks **x 3 sets** in total
20 seconds rest between sets

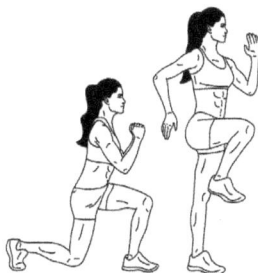

10 lunge step-ups **x 3 sets** in total
20 seconds rest between sets

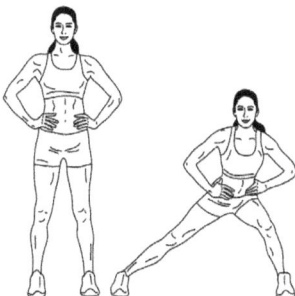

20 side lunges **x 3 sets** in total
20 seconds rest between sets

4. Abs

Strong abs help you stand, walk, run and jump better. They improve posture, prevent fatigue and augment physical performance.

Develop strong abs to help you level up in your physical abilities.

Athena's PLAYBOOK

Day 4 | Abs

no sets | keep the plank
throughout
the sequence

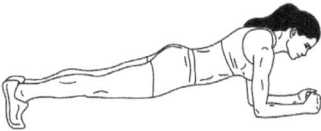

30sec elbow plank

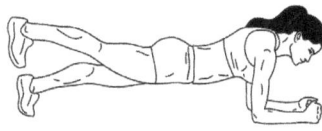

30sec raised leg elbow plank
15 seconds per leg

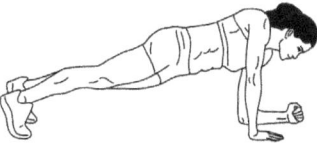

30sec uneven plank
15 seconds per side

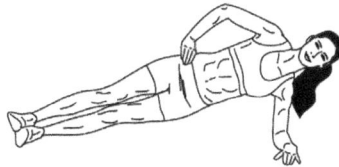

60sec side elbow plank
30 seconds per side

5. Cardio

Cardiovascular fitness preserves biological youthfulness and helps the body be more energetic and durable. It is also good for overall brain health as it helps with oxygen content in the bloodstream at the blood/ brain interface plus, it really helps establish good lung health.

Athena's PLAYBOOK

© darebee.com

Day 5 | Cardio

Level I 3 sets
Level II 5 sets
Level III 7 sets

2 minutes rest between sets

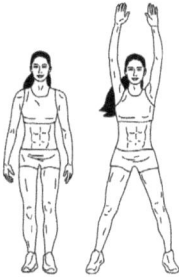

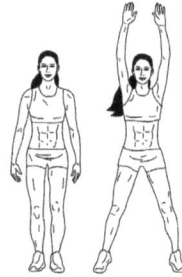

20 jumping jacks

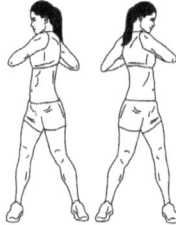

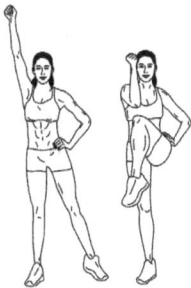

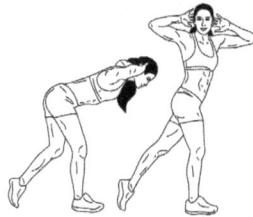

4 twists

20 jumping jacks

4 knee-to-elbows

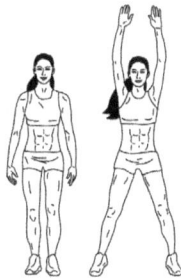

20 jumping jacks

4 deadlift & twist

6. Yoga

Flexibility is key to achieving full range of motion in your muscles and joints. It can help prevent injury, aid muscle recovery and even help build better quality of muscle overall. Yoga poses help establish a good range of motion and aid in the flexibility of joints and the spine.

Athena's PLAYBOOK

© darebee.com

Day 6 | Yoga

Hold each pose for 20 seconds then move on to the next one. Repeat the sequence again on the other side.

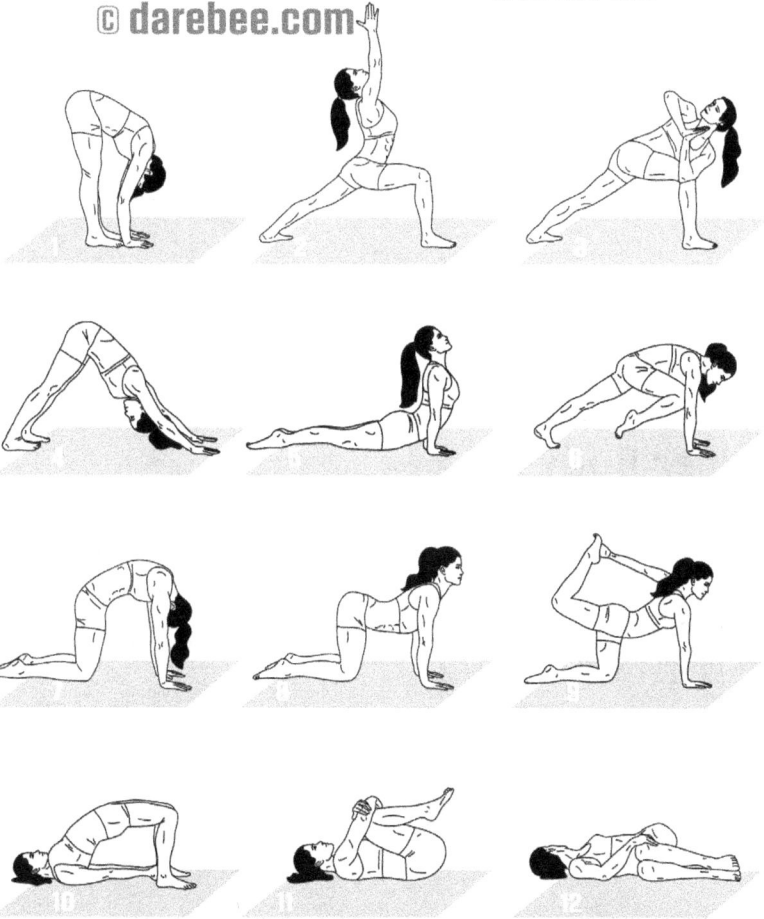

7. Upper Body

Upper body strength is important for a whole range of everyday tasks. It also helps us establish our athletic ability in a wide variety of physical activities and sports. Developing upper body strength requires a consistent approach to training.

Athena's PLAYBOOK

© darebee.com

Day 7
Upper Body

2 minutes rest
between exercises

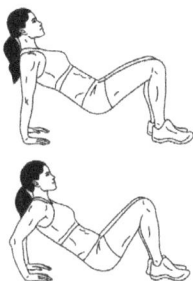

10 tricep dips **x 3 sets** in total
20 seconds rest between sets

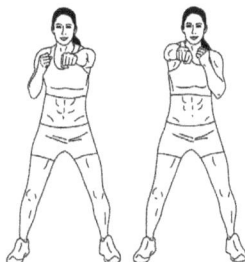

40 punches **x 3 sets** in total
20 seconds rest between sets

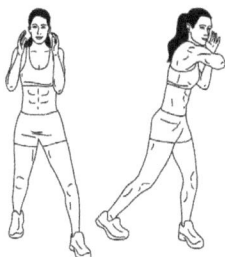

10 elbow strikes **x 3 sets** in total
20 seconds rest between sets

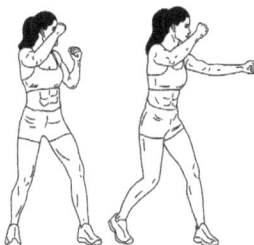

40 backfists **x 3 sets** in total
20 seconds rest between sets

8. Lower Body

Lower body strength is also important for a whole range of everyday tasks. It also helps us establish our athletic ability in a wide variety of physical activities and sports. Lower body strength increases our overall power output by driving the performance of upper body activities such as boxing or sports that require good hand/eye coordination. Developing good lower body strength also requires a consistent approach to training.

Athena's PLAYBOOK
© darebee.com

Day 8 | Lower Body

Level I 3 sets
Level II 4 sets
Level III 5 sets

2 minutes rest between sets

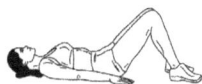

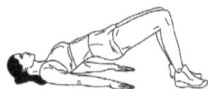

20 bridges

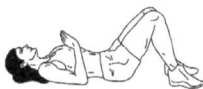

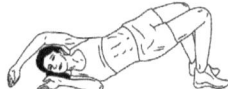

10 bridge taps

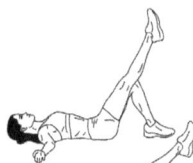

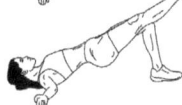

10 single leg bridges

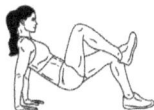

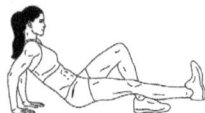

20 push kicks

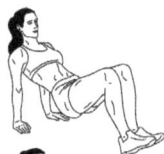

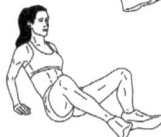

10 butterfly dips

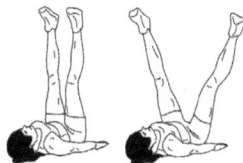

10 V-extensions

9. Cardio

Technically, cardio refers to cardiovascular health. Exercises that help improve the body's circulatory system function are good cardio exercises. The body's cardiovascular system is made up of the heart and the body's network of capillaries, arteries and blood vessels. Cardio workouts also exercise the lungs.

Athena's PLAYBOOK

© darebee.com

Day 9 | Cardio

Level I 3 sets
Level II 5 sets
Level III 7 sets

2 minutes rest between sets

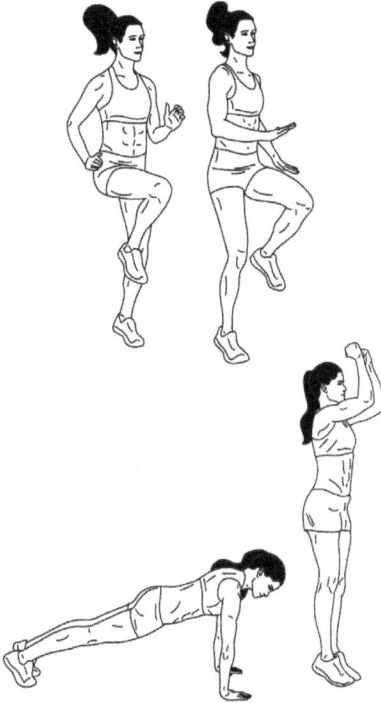

20 high knees

2 basic burpees w / jump

20 high knees

2 basic burpees w / jump

20 high knees

2 basic burpees w / jump

20 high knees

2 basic burpees w / jump

20 high knees

2 basic burpees w / jump

done

10. Upper Body

To develop good upper body strength requires exercise that utilizes a combination of open and closed-chain kinetics. The Athena's Playbook program makes good use of both providing a balanced approach that makes itself felt by the end of the program.

Athena's PLAYBOOK
© darebee.com

Day 10 | Upper Body

Level I 3 sets
Level II 4 sets
Level III 5 sets

2 minutes rest between sets

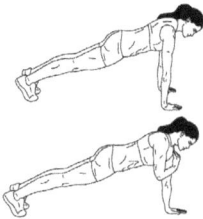

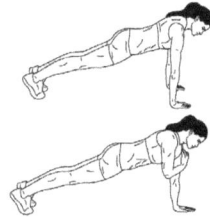

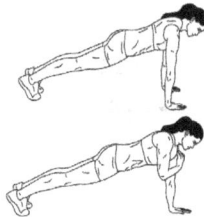

6 shoulder taps

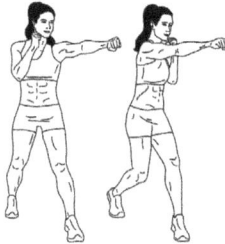

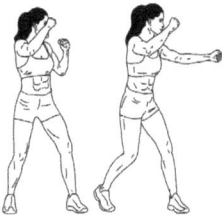

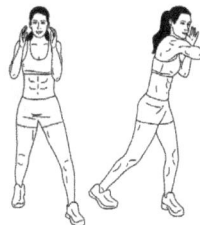

20 punches

6 shoulder taps

20 backfists

6 shoulder taps

20 elbow strikes

11. Lower Body

Good lower body strength doesn't just need strong quads and calves. It also requires powerful glutes, strong front hip flexors and powerful side hip flexors. Training the tendons and ligaments that form part of the body's lower system delivers physical power when you need it.

Athena's PLAYBOOK
© darebee.com

Day 11
Lower Body
2 minutes rest between exercises

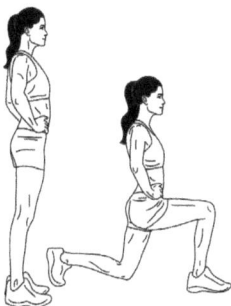

20 lunges **x 3 sets** in total
20 seconds rest between sets

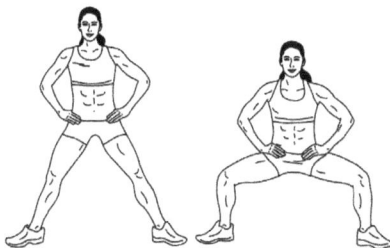

20 wide squats **x 3 sets** in total
20 seconds rest between sets

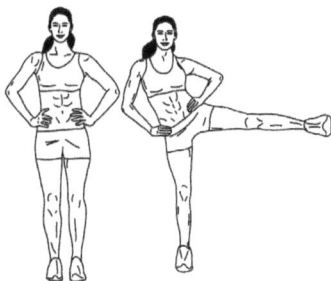

20 side leg raises **x 3 sets** in total
20 seconds rest between sets

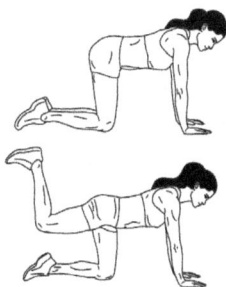

20 donkey kicks **x 3 sets** in total
20 seconds rest between sets

12. Abs

Strong abs help your body sit, stand, walk, run and jump better. They help improve posture and help reduce the loss of physical power as the body transfers energy from its lower system to its upper one. Pretty much every physical activity we engage in requires strong abs.

Athena's PLAYBOOK

Day 12 | Abs

Level I   2 sets
Level II 3 sets
Level III 4 sets

2 minutes rest between sets

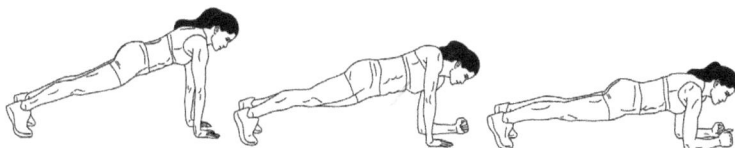

10 up and down planks

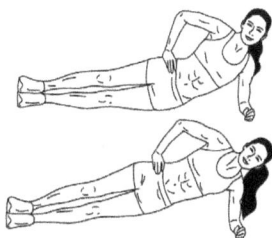

20 side bridges

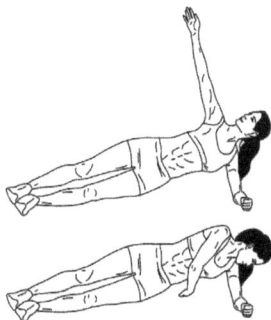

20 side plank rotations

13. Cardio

Regular cardio workouts help strengthen all five components of the body's cardiovascular system: the heart, blood vessels, arteries, capillaries and blood veins. Each of these has a specialized way of operating though all together function to produce a highly oxygenated state of being that allows us to perform demanding physical functions.

Athena's PLAYBOOK

Day 13 | Cardio

Level I 3 sets
Level II 5 sets
Level III 7 sets

2 minutes rest between sets

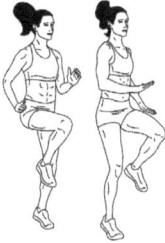

20 high knees

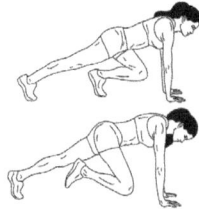

4 climbers

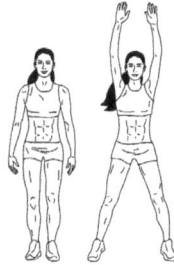

20 jumping jacks

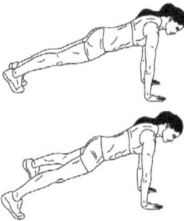

4 plank jacks

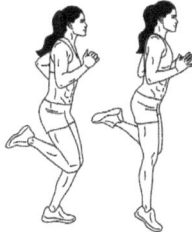

20 butt-kicks

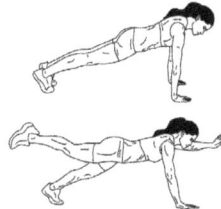

4 alt arm / leg raises

14. Combat

Combat moves are always a challenge. They demand strength, coordination, flexibility, agility and endurance. The benefits however are incredible. They help develop cardiovascular and aerobic fitness, maintain youthful muscles and, according to studies, increased mental alertness.

Athena's PLAYBOOK

© darebee.com

Day 14 | Combat

Level I 3 sets
Level II 5 sets
Level III 7 sets

2 minutes rest between sets

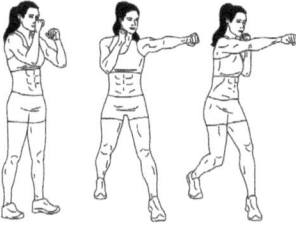

20combos jab + cross

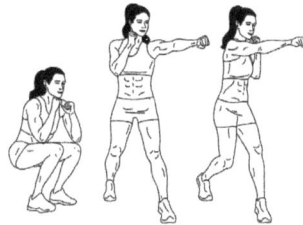

20combos squat + jab + cross

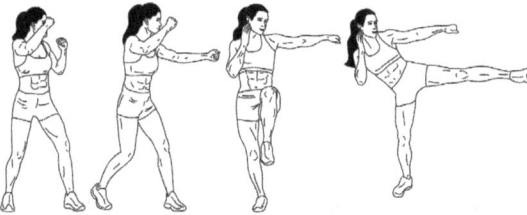

20combos backfist + side kick

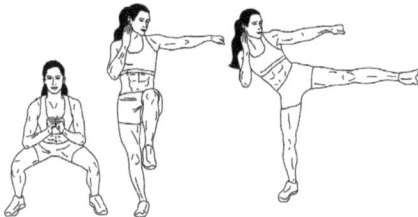

20combos squat + side kick

15. Yoga

Yoga exercises that help develop the flexibility of the spine and pelvis free the body's range of movement and increase its athletic capabilities. They also incease blood flow and tissue health in regions that would normally not get a lot of stimulation.

Athena's PLAYBOOK
@darebee.com

Day 15 | Yoga

Hold each pose for 20 seconds then move on to the next one. Repeat the sequence again on the other side.

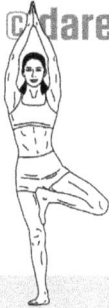

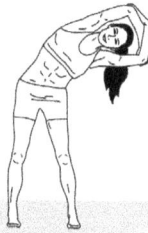

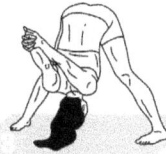

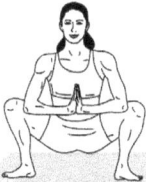

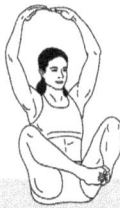

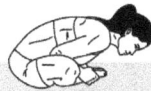

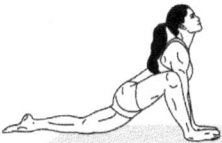

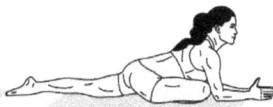

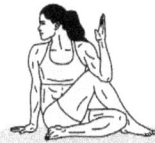

16. Upper Body

Punching is an open kinetic chain exercise that challenges the aerobic and cardiovascular systems of the body, helps develop limb speed and lower/upper body coordination. Planks help develop a strong core that increase the body's overall capacity to produce powerful movement.

Athena's PLAYBOOK
© darebee.com

Day 16 | Upper Body

Level I 3 sets
Level II 5 sets
Level III 7 sets

2 minutes rest between sets

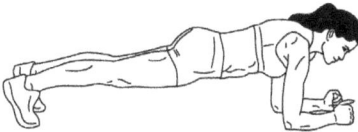

10-count plank hold

20 punches

10-count plank hold

20 punches

10-count plank hold

20 punches

10-count plank hold

20 punches

done

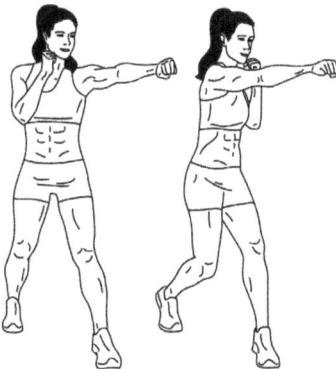

17. Lower Body

Dynamic, lower body exercises help develop explosive strength and good joint stability. Hip flexor exercises allow the lower body to reduce the load felt by the joints and maintain endurance and power without tiring.

Athena's PLAYBOOK

© darebee.com

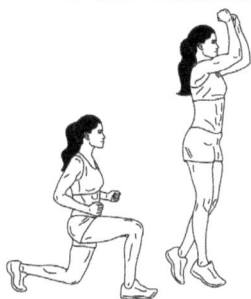

10 jumping lunges **x 4 sets** in total
2 sets left side / 2 sets right side
20 seconds rest between sets

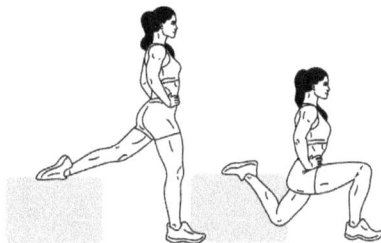

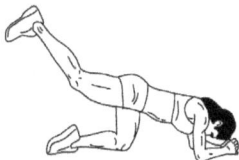

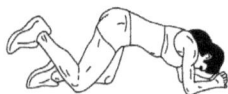

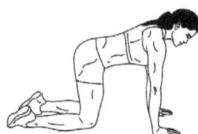

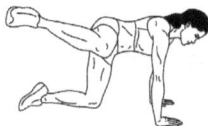

10 split squats **x 4 sets** in total
2 sets left side / 2 sets right side
20 seconds rest between sets

20 back kicks **x 4 sets** in total
2 sets left side / 2 sets right side
20 seconds rest between sets

20 side leg lifts **x 4 sets** in total
2 sets left side / 2 sets right side
20 seconds rest between sets

18. Cardio

Cardio exercises don't just make you sweat, they also train the connective tissue in the body (called fascia) and help you feel that you are in overall control of what your body can do. By now you should begin to feel the progression effect in the exercises of this program; and be in greater control of your body.

Athena's PLAYBOOK

© darebee.com

Day 18 | Cardio

Level I   3 sets
Level II 5 sets
Level III 7 sets

2 minutes rest between sets

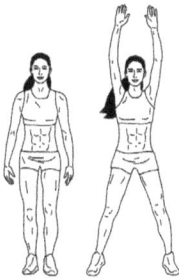

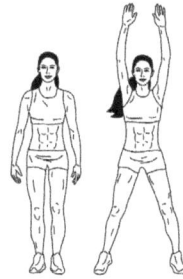

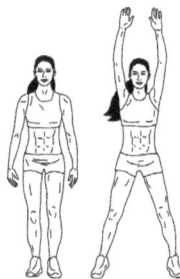

20 jumping jacks

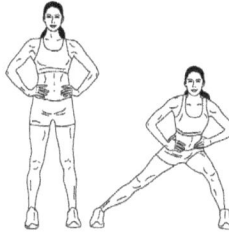

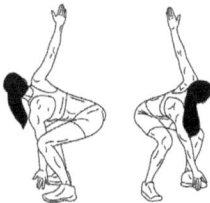

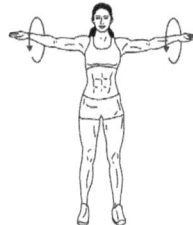

4 side lunges

20 jumping jacks

4 windmills

20 jumping jacks

20 raised arm circles

19. Tendon Strength

Tendons allow the muscles to unleash their full power, they help make physical movement easier and they provide joint stability that safeguards against injury. Strengthening the tendons requires patience and perseverance. They respond slower than muscles but tend to also lose their strength slower during periods of inactivity.

Athena's PLAYBOOK

© darebee.com

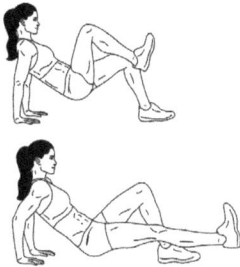

40 push kicks **x 2 sets** in total
1 set left side / 1 set right side
20 seconds rest between sets

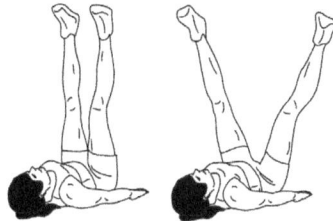

20 V-extensions **x 2 sets** in total
1 set left side / 1 set right side
20 seconds rest between sets

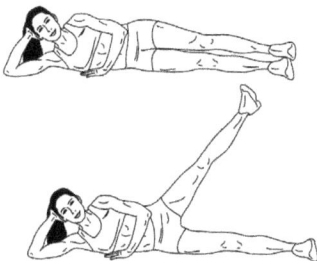

40 side leg raises **x 2 sets** in total
1 set left side / 1 set right side
20 seconds rest between sets

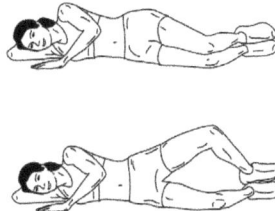

20 clamshells **x 2 sets** in total
1 set left side / 1 set right side
20 seconds rest between sets

20. Abs

Strong abs help support the back and spine better. They help build physical endurance by reducing the vibrations that core and back muscles feel during impact exercise. This resists the build-up of fatigue and delivers a stronger physical performance. Strong abs also help develop a better, overall posture and a better sense of control.

Athena's PLAYBOOK

© darebee.com

Day 20 | Abs

no sets | keep the plank throughout the sequence

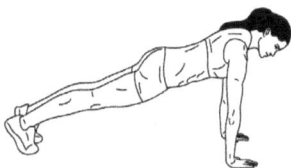

20sec plank

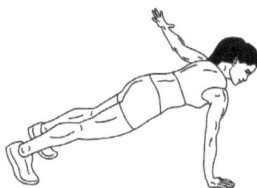

40sec one arm plank
20 seconds per arm

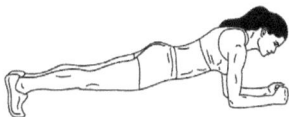

20sec elbow plank

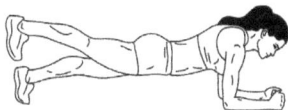

20sec raised leg elbow plank
10 seconds per leg

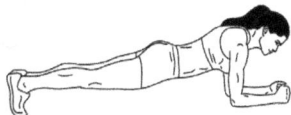

40sec elbow plank

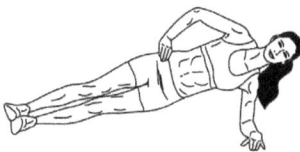

40sec side elbow plank
20 seconds per side

21. Combat

Combat moves recruit virtually all of the body's muscles and utilize both the cardiovascular and aerobic systems. This makes them perfect for those who want to achieve fast improvements in balance, speed, coordination and physical power. They also provide the best way possible to detox from stress and anxiety and find that inner peace.

Athena's PLAYBOOK

© darebee.com

Day 21 | Combat

Level I 3 sets
Level II 5 sets
Level III 7 sets

2 minutes rest between sets

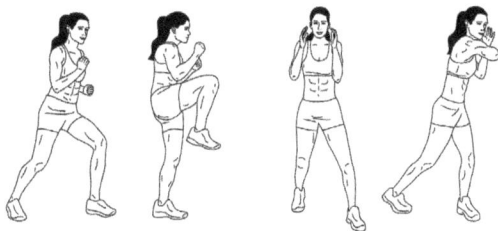

20combos knee strike + elbow strike

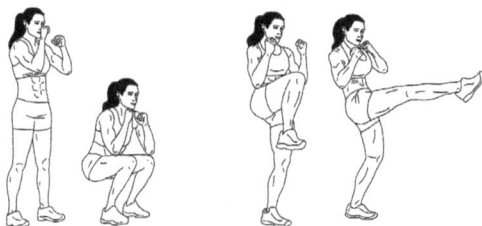

20combos squats + front kick

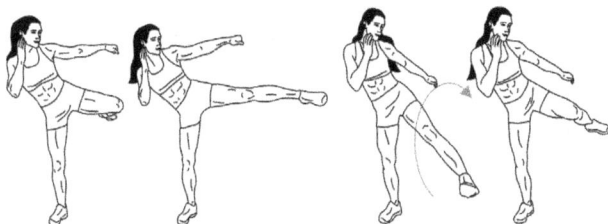

20combos turning kick + hook kick

22. Upper Body

Upper body strength is developed through the sustained application of exercises that trigger the body's adaptive response. Arms, shoulders and chest are alos used to balance the body when the lower body's muscles get to work. This workout has a little bit of everything but the focus is on the upper body.

Athena's PLAYBOOK

© darebee.com

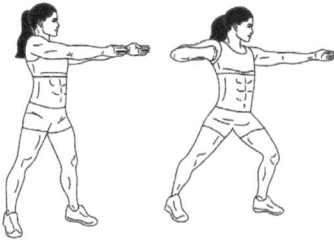

20 archers **x 4 sets** in total
20 seconds rest between sets

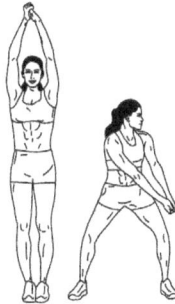

20 cross chops **x 4 sets** in total
20 seconds rest between sets

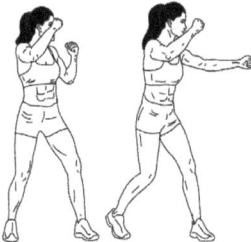

20 backfists **x 4 sets** in total
20 seconds rest between sets

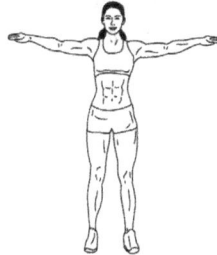

5 minutes raised arm hold

23. Yoga

Yoga delivers a number of physical, emotional and psychological benefits. Calmness, lower stress levels, deeper breathing, flexibility, balance and improved cardiovascular function are just some of them.

Athena's PLAYBOOK

© darebee.com

Day 23 | Yoga

Hold each pose for 20 seconds then move on to the next one. Repeat the sequence again on the other side.

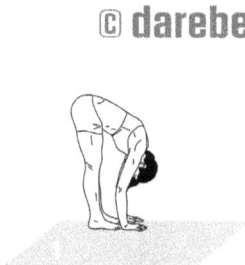

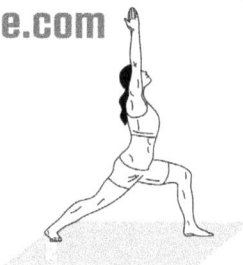

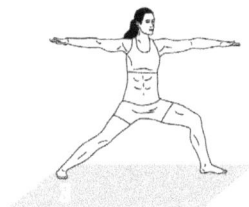

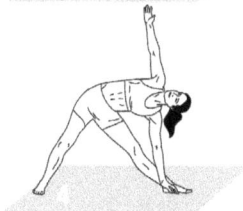

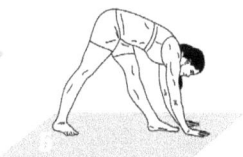

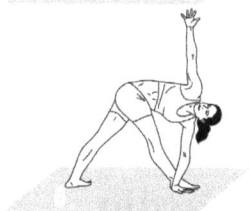

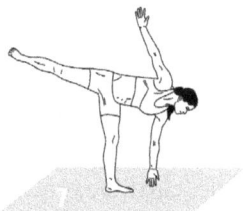

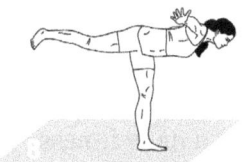

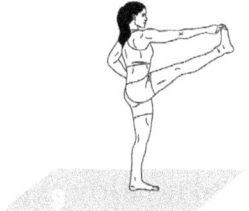

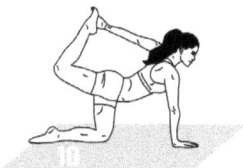

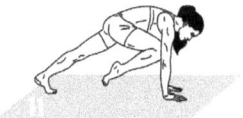

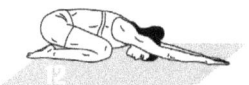

24. Cardio

Cardio workouts help develop a robust cardiovascular system that helps the pulmonary cycle that connects the heart with the lungs, enrich blood oxygen levels and help maintain metabolic functions and brain health. Practised regularly, as part of a daily fitness routine, cardio exercise helps build faster physical responses to the demands of increased physical activity.

Athena's PLAYBOOK

Day 24 | Cardio

Level I   3 sets
Level II 5 sets
Level III 7 sets

2 minutes rest between sets

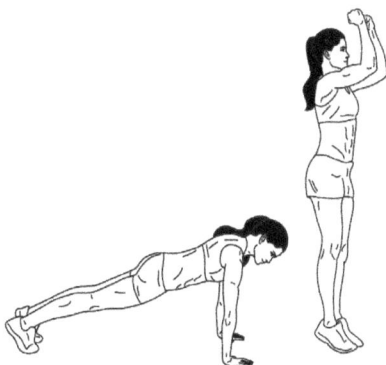

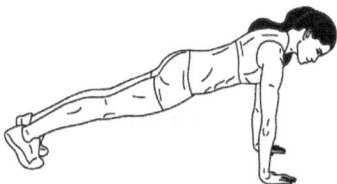

5 basic burpees w / jump

10-count plank hold

5 basic burpees w / jump

10-count plank hold

5 basic burpees w / jump

10-count plank hold

5 basic burpees w / jump

10-count plank hold

5 basic burpees w / jump

10-count plank hold

done

25. Lower Body

Lower body exercises that focus on the development of specific muscle groups can deliver faster results, over time, that help amplify the body's physical power.

Many lower body exercises do not require particularly complex exercise routines or specialized equipment.

Athena's PLAYBOOK

Day 25
Lower Body

2 minutes rest between exercises

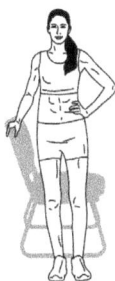

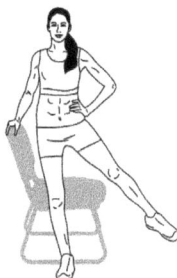

50 side leg raises **x 4 sets** in total
2 sets left leg / 2 sets right leg
20 seconds rest between sets

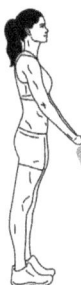

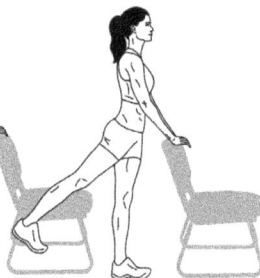

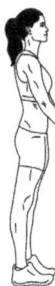

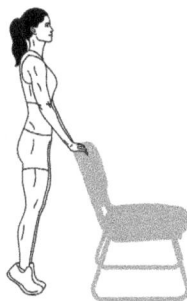

50 back leg raises **x 4 sets** in total
2 sets left leg / 2 sets right leg
20 seconds rest between sets

30 calf raises **x 3 sets** in total
20 seconds rest between sets

26. Abs

Abs respond quickly to exercise and lose their strength comparatively slowly in relation to other muscle groups. All the more reason to work on them on a regular basis, helping maintain their strength and capability.

Athena's PLAYBOOK

© darebee.com

Day 26 | Abs

Level I 2 sets
Level II 3 sets
Level III 4 sets

2 minutes rest between sets

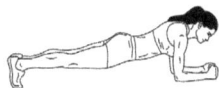

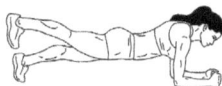

10 plank leg raises

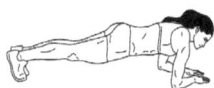

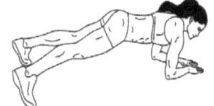

10 plank side-step

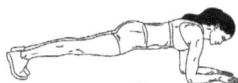

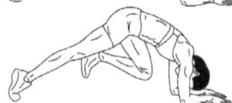

10 plank knee-ins

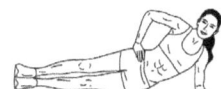

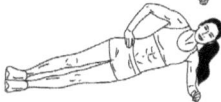

10 side bridges

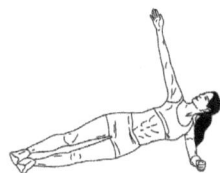

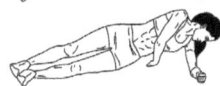

10 side plank rotations

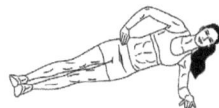

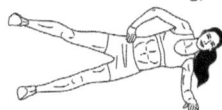

10 side plank leg raises

27. Upper Body

Upper body strength requires persistence and structure. Frequent upper body workouts are key to triggering the body's adaptive response which then delivers gains in strength and conditioning.

Athena's PLAYBOOK

Day 27 | Upper Body

Level I   3 sets
Level II 5 sets
Level III 7 sets

2 minutes rest between sets

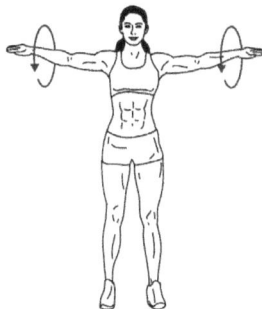

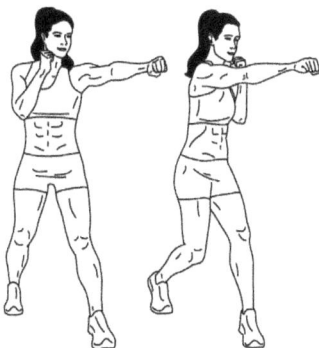

Keep your arms up:

10 raised arm circles

20 punches

10 raised arm circles

20 punches

10 raised arm circles

20 punches

10 raised arm circles

20 punches

done

28. Lower Body

Lower body strength requires the activation of the body's lower kinetic chain. This always brings about neurobiological and mechanical changes that manifest themselves, over time, in greater strength, stability and control.

Athena's PLAYBOOK

© darebee.com

Day 28 | Lower Body

Level I 3 sets
Level II 4 sets
Level III 5 sets

2 minutes rest between sets

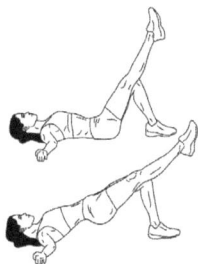

20 single leg bridges

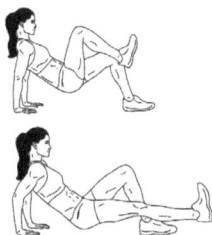

20 push kicks

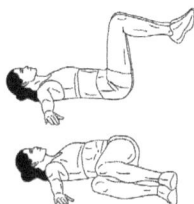

10 half wipers

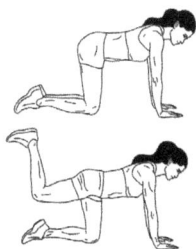

20 donkey kicks

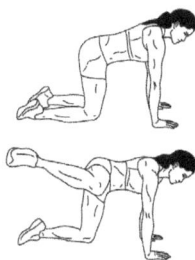

20 side leg lifts

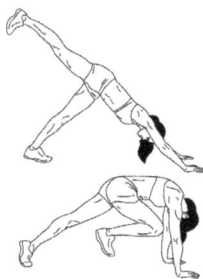

10 knee-in back kicks

29. Cardio

Good cardio exercises activate the cardiovascular system and get the heart and lungs working alongside the body's circulatory system. Day 29 of this month-long program will get your body temperature up and your breathing going.

Athena's PLAYBOOK

Day 29 | Cardio

Level I 3 sets
Level II 5 sets
Level III 7 sets

2 minutes rest between sets

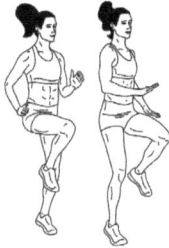
20 high knees

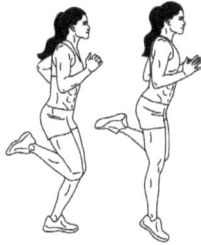
10 butt kicks

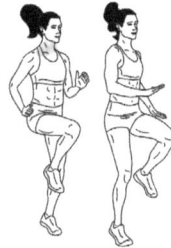
20 high knees

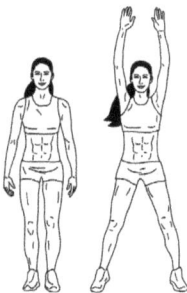
10 jumping jacks

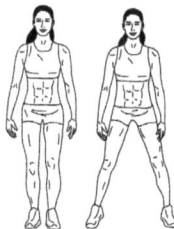
20 half jacks

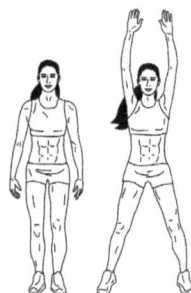
10 jumping jacks

30. Combat

Combat moves are always a challenge. The complex moves require agility, flexibility, balance and coordination. They engage the power of both the body and brain. This last day of the 30-day set is a test. Get through it at Level III with EC and you've reached the pinnacle of Athena's playbook.

Athena's PLAYBOOK

© darebee.com

Day 30 | Combat

Level I   3 sets
Level II 5 sets
Level III 7 sets

2 minutes rest between sets

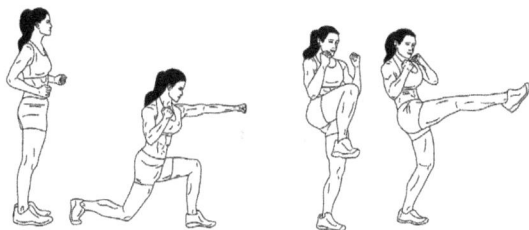

20combos lunge punch + front kick

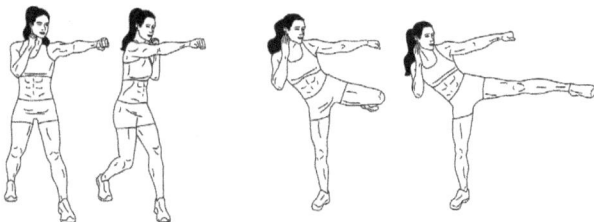

20combos jab + cross + turning kick

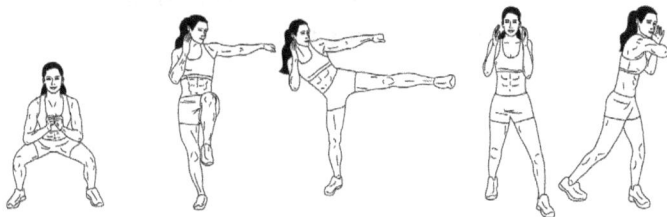

20combos squat + side kick + elbow strike

Balance the body - Challenge the mind

Throughout the Athena's Playbook program you engage in exercises that challenge your body and brain. Ultimately, of course, the brain is central to everything. Without developing specific neural pathways it becomes hard to control the body in specific ways and it even becomes hard to take full advantage of the power the body's muscles can generate.

So you need a strong, healthy mind to achieve a strong, healthy body.

What we know now of the mind/body divide shows that there is no mind/body divide. Neural pathways extend throughout the body. There are clusters of neurons processing information and acting like a mini-brain in the stomach and the heart. The brain is reliant on the health of the heart, the lungs and the vascular system to function properly.

We truly cannot hope to train one part of us without training the other. More than that, even within the domain of the brain and the domain of the body systems seem to rely on connectivity, the network effect and overlapping connections, to work.

The body's kinetic chains is an example of this as well as the brain's call on different centers that help it synthesize what we understand as cognition.

What all this means is that as you do 'simple' workouts you improve the function of your brain. As the function of your brain improves, the workings of your body also improve.

The benefits of Yoga exercises

Neuroscientific studies have shown that yoga changes specific structures of the brain and has the same benefits as aerobics on the body.

More specifically, the amygdala, a brain structure that contributes to emotional regulation, tends to be larger in yoga practitioners than in their peers who do not practice yoga. The prefrontal cortex, cingulate cortex and brain networks such as the default mode network also tend to be larger or more efficient in those who regularly practice yoga.

In the pages that follow you will get the chance to incorporate regular yoga workouts in your lifestyle. On each page you will also learn something new about the health benefits of yoga exercises.

1. Balance

Benefits of improved balance:

- Improved posture
- Stronger core
- Improved physical performance
- Faster cognitive functions due to improved circulation
- Injury prevention

30 days of
YOGA
Day 1
© darebee.com

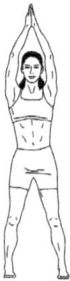

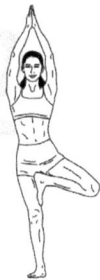

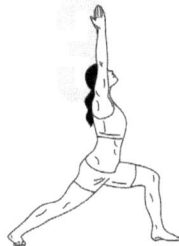

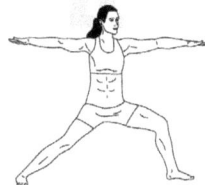

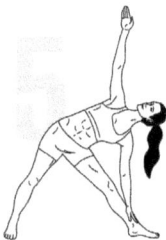

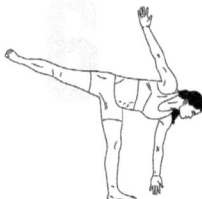

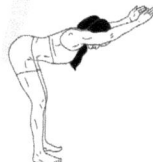

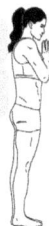

Hold each pose for 20 seconds then move on to the next one.
Repeat the sequence again on the other side.

2. Spine Health

Benefits of a healthy spine:

- Better posture
- Resistance to fatigue
- Agility
- Greater power
- Improved balance

30 days of
YOGA
Day 2
© darebee.com

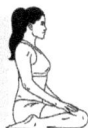

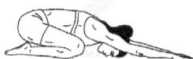

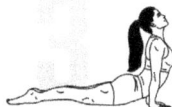

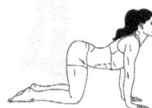

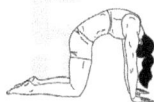

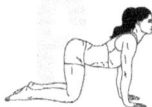

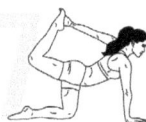

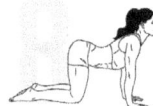

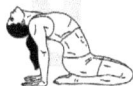

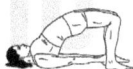

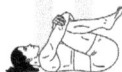

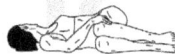

Hold each pose for 20 seconds then move on to the next one.
Repeat the sequence again on the other side.

3. Brain Health

Benefits of meditation:

- Stress management
- Emotional regulation
- Improved focus
- Increased patience
- Increased self-awareness

30 days of
YOGA

Day 3
© darebee.com

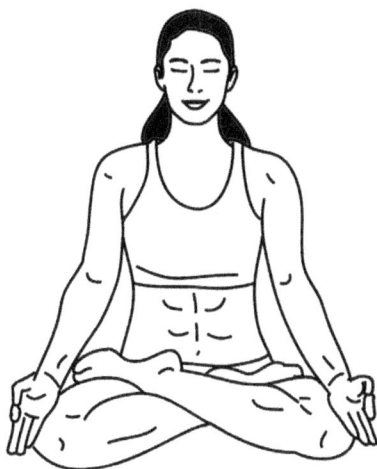

5 minutes
meditation

4. Agility

Benefits of agility include:

- Improved balance
- Greater flexibility
- More control
- Better posture
- Better body placement

30 days of
YOGA

Day 4

© darebee.com

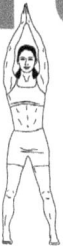

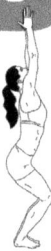

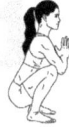

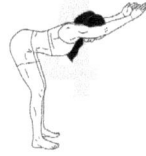

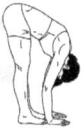

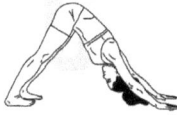

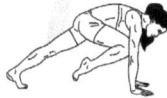

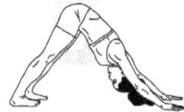

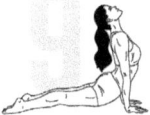

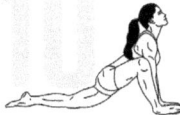

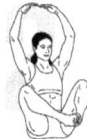

Hold each pose for 20 seconds then move on to the next one.
Repeat the sequence again on the other side.

5. Neck and Spine Health

Benefits of a strong, healthy neck and spine:

- Agility
- Improved posture
- Better coordination
- Improved focus when running
- Improved body placement when jumping

30 days of
YOGA

Day 5

© darebee.com

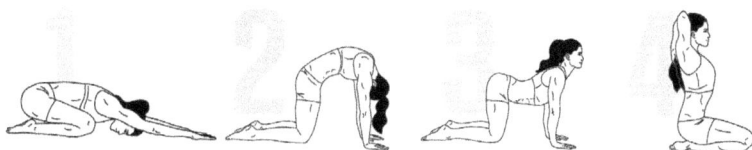

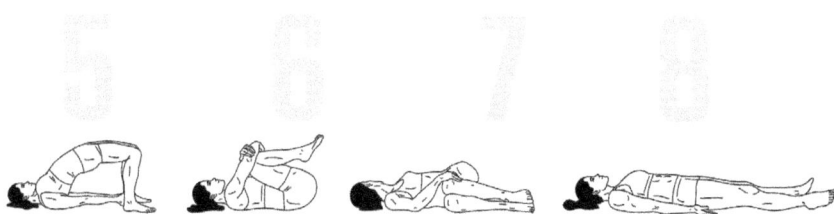

Hold each pose for 20 seconds then move on to the next one.
Repeat the sequence again on the other side.

6. Meditation

Benefits of meditation include:

- Improved concentration
- Reduced anxiety
- Better emotional regulation
- Reduced stress
- Improved physical and mental wellbeing

30 days of
YOGA

Day 6
© darebee.com

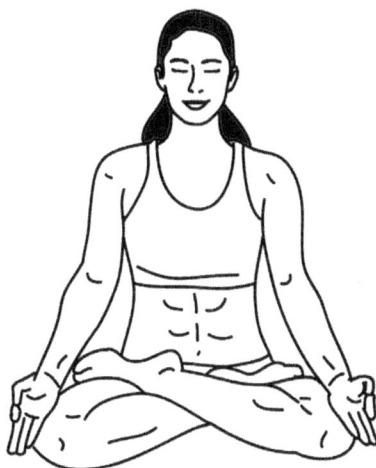

5 minutes
meditation

7. Flexibility

Health benefits of flexibility:

- Fewer injuries
- Greater freedom of movement
- Agility
- Stronger muscles
- Greater speed

30 days of
YOGA
Day 7
© darebee.com

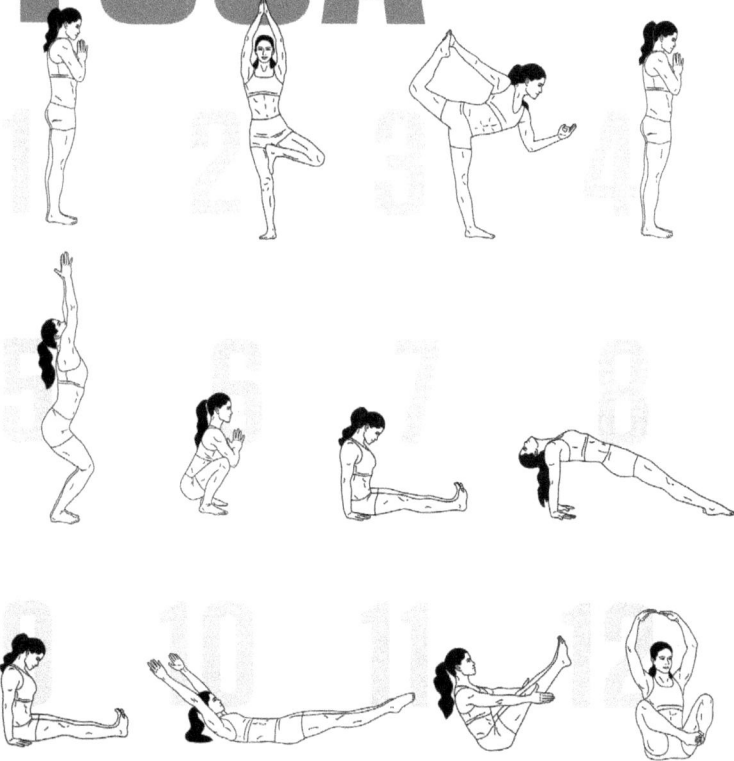

Hold each pose for 20 seconds then move on to the next one.
Repeat the sequence again on the other side.

8. Suppleness

Benefits of being supple:

- Faster movements
- Greater balance
- More power
- Precision
- Agility

30 days of
YOGA
Day 8
© darebee.com

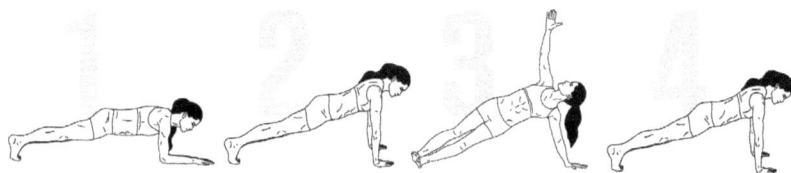

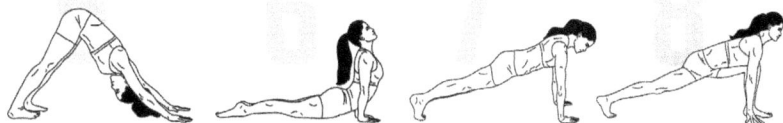

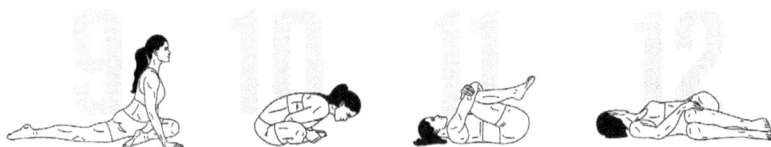

Hold each pose for 20 seconds then move on to the next one.
Repeat the sequence again on the other side.

9. Meditation

Benefits of meditation include:

- Improved concentration
- Reduced anxiety
- Better emotional regulation
- Reduced stress
- Improved physical and mental wellbeing

30 days of
YOGA

Day 9
© darebee.com

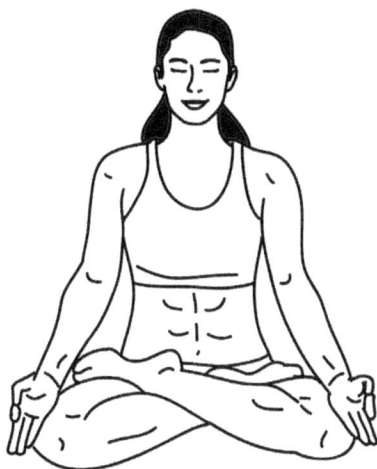

5 minutes
meditation

10. Stability

Health benefits of stability:

- Improved mobility
- Fewer chances of injury
- Better balance
- Improved coordination
- Stronger lower body joints

30 days of
YOGA
Day 10
© darebee.com

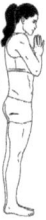

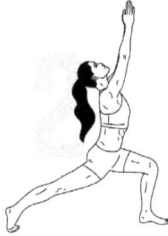

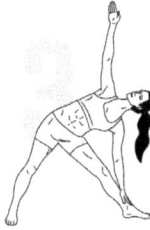

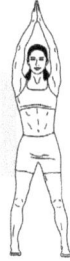

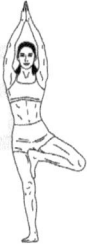

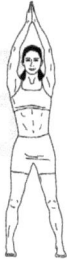

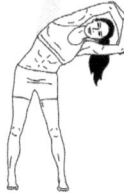

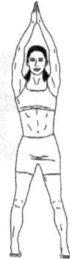

Hold each pose for 20 seconds then move on to the next one.
Repeat the sequence again on the other side.

11. Spinal strength

Health benefits of spinal strength:

- Improved posture
- Reduced lower back aches
- Better agility
- Greater power
- Improved flexibility

30 days of
YOGA
Day 11
© darebee.com

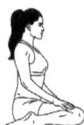

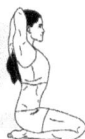

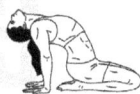

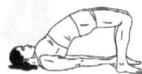

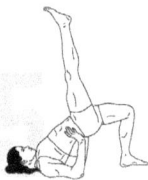

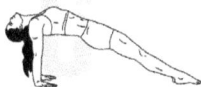

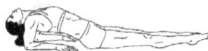

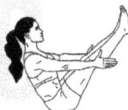

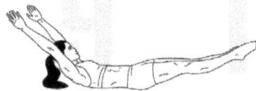

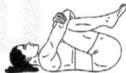

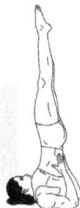

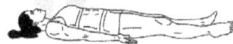

Hold each pose for 20 seconds then move on to the next one.
Repeat the sequence again on the other side.

12. Meditation

Health benefits of prolonged meditation:

- Improved cognitive function
- Reduced stress and anxiety
- Improved mental focus
- Improved concentration on tasks
- Overall, better physical and mental health

30 days of
YOGA

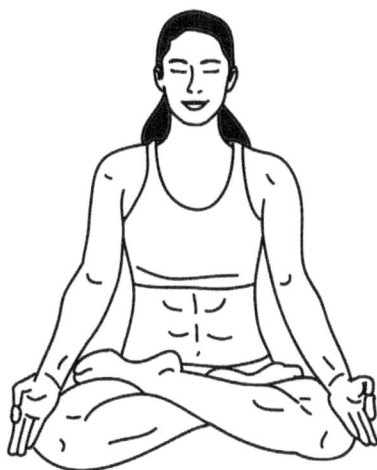

Day 12
© darebee.com

10 minutes
meditation

13. Harmony

Health benefits of harmonic physical movements:

- Better balance
- Greater agility
- Improved coordination
- Better joint strength and stability
- Improved cardiovascular function

30 days of
YOGA

Day 13
© darebee.com

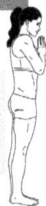

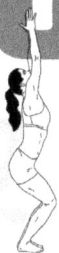

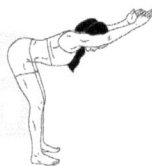

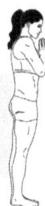

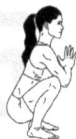

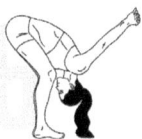

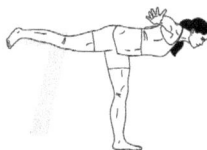

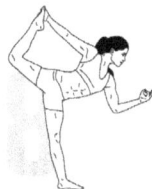

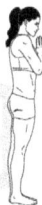

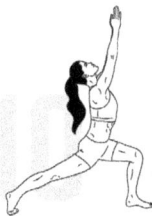

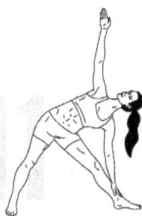

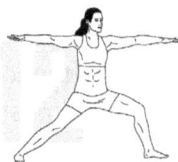

Hold each pose for 20 seconds then move on to the next one.
Repeat the sequence again on the other side.

14. Spinal Stretching

Health benefits of spinal stretching:

- Improved blood flow to extremeties
- Greater freedom of motion in the body
- Improved posture and neck strength
- Reduced experience of lower back pain
- Improved hip joint health and stability

30 days of
YOGA
Day 14

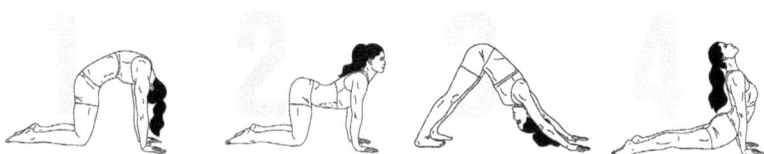

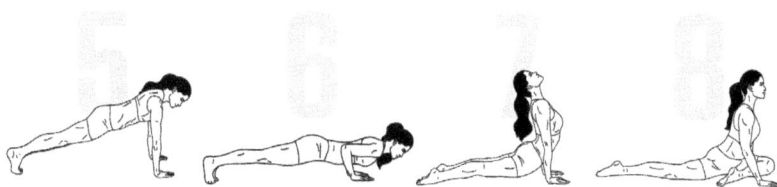

Hold each pose for 20 seconds then move on to the next one.
Repeat the sequence again on the other side.

15. Meditation

Health benefits of prolonged meditation:

- Improved cognitive function
- Reduced stress and anxiety
- Improved mental focus
- Improved concentration on tasks
- Overall, better physical and mental health

30 days of
YOGA

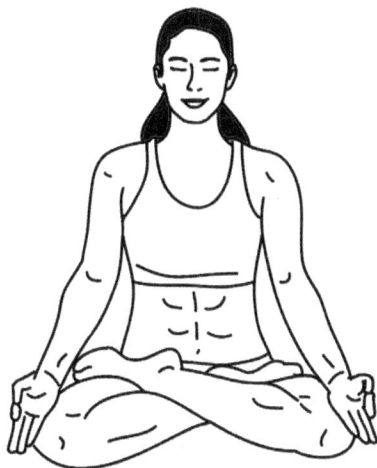

10 minutes
meditation

16. Lower Body Flexibility

Health benefits of lower body flexibility:

- Improved lower body movement
- Greater coordination and balance
- An increase in physical power
- Improved blood flow through pelvic region
- Younger, more flexible lower body joints

30 days of
YOGA

Day 16
© darebee.com

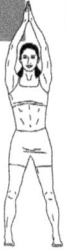

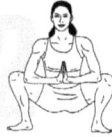

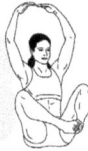

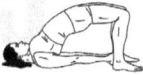

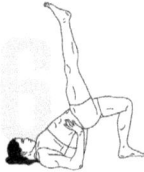

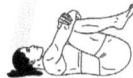

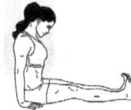

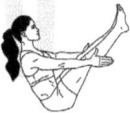

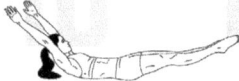

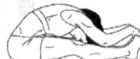

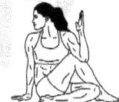

Hold each pose for 20 seconds then move on to the next one.
Repeat the sequence again on the other side.

17. Spine Health

Health benefits of greater spine health:

- Improved agility
- Better balance and posture
- Improved athletic performance
- Reduction in chances for injury
- Improved sense of physical wellbeing

30 days of
YOGA
Day 17
© darebee.com

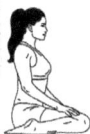 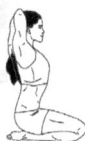 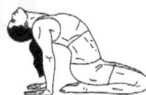 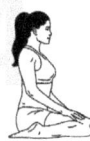

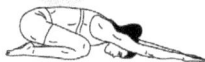 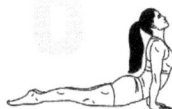 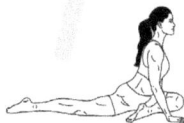

Hold each pose for 20 seconds then move on to the next one.
Repeat the sequence again on the other side.

18. Meditation

Health benefits of regular meditation:

- Improved mood control
- Greater emotional stability
- Greater control over stress and anxiety
- Improved sense of psychological wellbeing
- Greater self-awareness and better sense of purpose

30 days of
YOGA

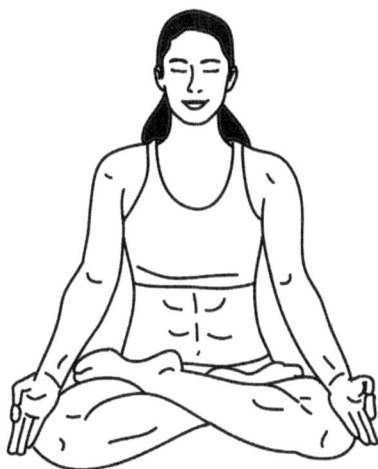

10 minutes
meditation

19. Balance

Health benefits of better balance:

- Improved posture
- Improved endurance
- Improved agility
- Improved flexibility
- Improved athleticism

30 days of
YOGA

Day 19

© darebee.com

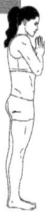

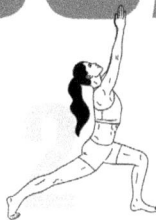

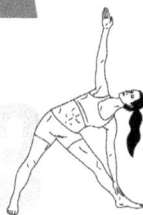

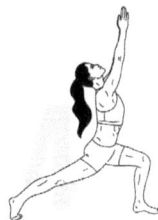

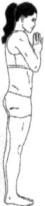

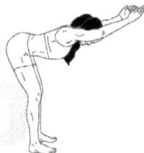

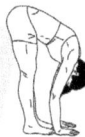

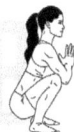

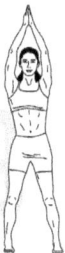

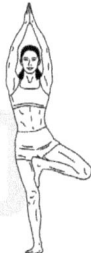

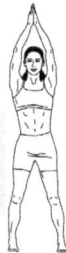

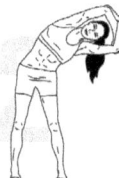

Hold each pose for 20 seconds then move on to the next one.
Repeat the sequence again on the other side.

20. Strength

Health benefits of improved strength:

- Resistance to fatigue
- Resistance to aging
- Improved immune system
- Improved cognitive functions
- Improved physical performance

30 days of
YOGA

Day 20
© darebee.com

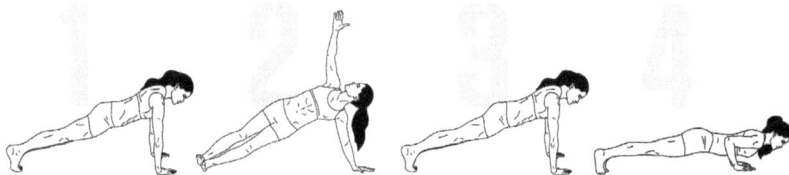

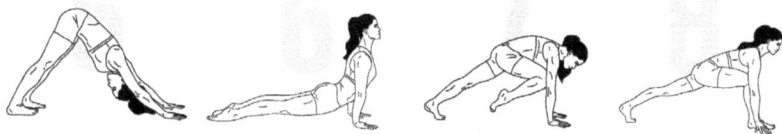

Hold each pose for 20 seconds then move on to the next one.
Repeat the sequence again on the other side.

21. Meditation

Health benefits of regular meditation:

- Improved mood control
- Greater emotional stability
- Greater control over stress and anxiety
- Improved sense of psychological wellbeing
- Greater self-awareness and better sense of purpose

30 days of
YOGA

Day 21
© darebee.com

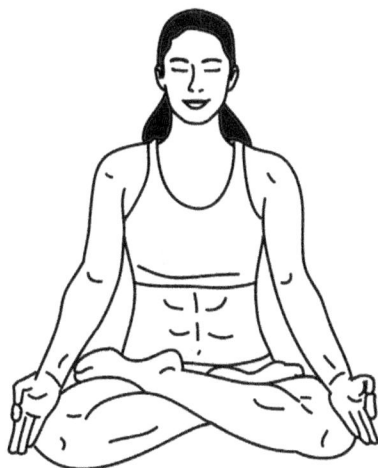

15 minutes
meditation

22. Strength & Flexibility

Health benefits of a strong, flexible body:

- Improved agility
- Better motor function
- Improved balance and power
- Fewer age-related aches and pains
- Resistance to illness and tiredness

30 days of
YOGA

Day 22
© darebee.com

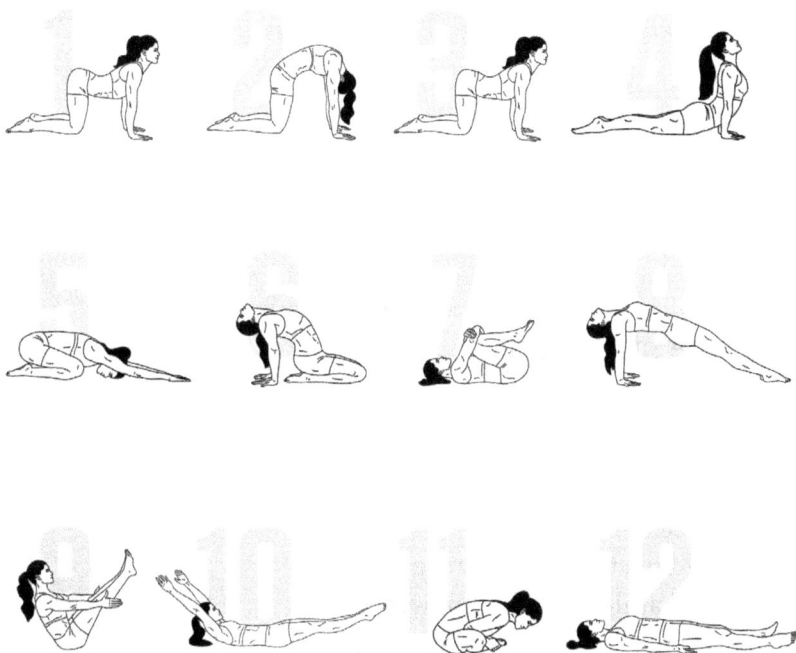

Hold each pose for 20 seconds then move on to the next one.
Repeat the sequence again on the other side.

23. Core stability

Health benefits of a strong core:

- Resistance to fatigue
- Improved posture and balance
- Improved athleticism and power
- More youthful attitude and demeanor
- A greater sense of control of body and mind

30 days of
YOGA

Day 23

© darebee.com

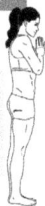

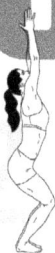

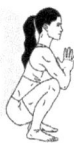

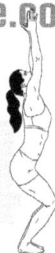

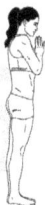

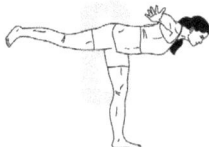

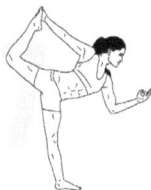

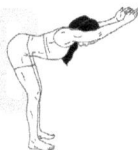

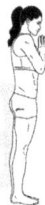

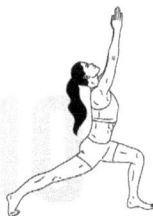

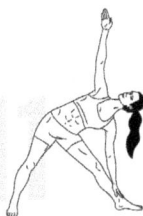

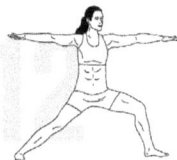

Hold each pose for 20 seconds then move on to the next one.
Repeat the sequence again on the other side.

24. Meditation

Health benefits of regular meditation:

- Enhanced emotional health
- Increased self-awareness
- Can combat addiction
- Longer attention span
- Improves memory

30 days of
YOGA

Day 24
© darebee.com

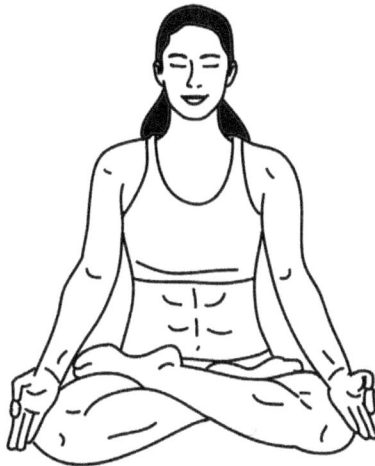

15 minutes
meditation

25. Flexibility

Health benefits of a flexible spine:

- Enhanced feelings of wellbeing
- Improved posture and movement
- Resistance to injury and physical fatigue
- Increased feeling of youthfulness and focus
- Better able to perform complex balance exercises

30 days of
YOGA

Day 25
© darebee.com

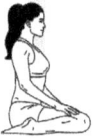

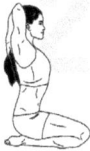

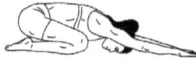

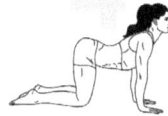

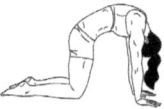

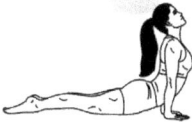

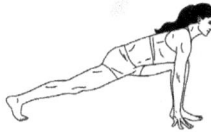

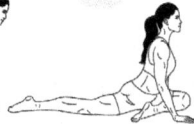

Hold each pose for 20 seconds then move on to the next one.
Repeat the sequence again on the other side.

26. Hips and Spine

Health benefits of a strong pelvic girdle:

- Improve bladder and bowel control
- Reduce the risk of prolapse
- Improve recovery from childbirth
- Improve recovery after prostate surgery (in men)
- Increase sexual sensation and orgasmic potential

30 days of
YOGA
Day 26
© darebee.com

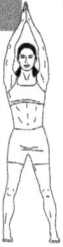

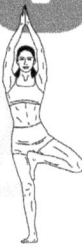

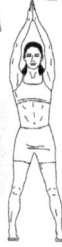

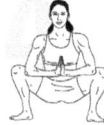

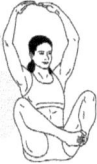

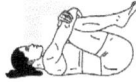

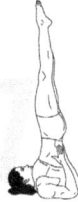

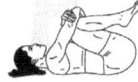

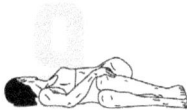

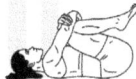

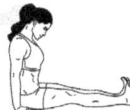

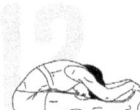

Hold each pose for 20 seconds then move on to the next one.
Repeat the sequence again on the other side.

27. Meditation

Health benefits of regular meditation:

- Enhanced emotional health
- Increased self-awareness
- Can combat addiction
- Longer attention span
- Improves memory

30 days of
YOGA

Day 27
© darebee.com

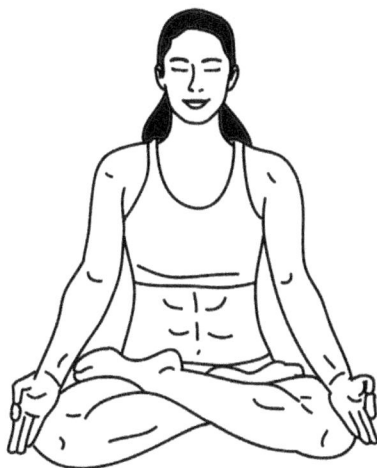

15 minutes
meditation

28. Agility

Health benefits of agility:

- Improved flexibility
- Better balance
- Greater muscle control
- Better muscle alignment
- Better posture during movement

30 days of
YOGA
Day 28
© darebee.com

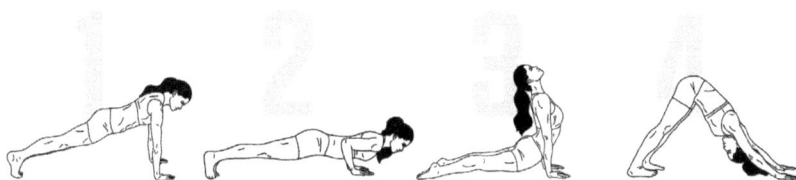

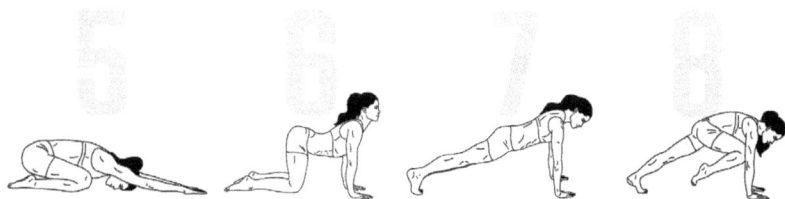

Hold each pose for 20 seconds then move on to the next one.
Repeat the sequence again on the other side.

29. Stability

Health benefits of greater stability:

- Better performance in weight-bearing activities
- Reduced chances of joint injury to the lower body
- Overall better athletic performance
- Greater resistance to muscle fatigue
- Better tendon/muscle coordination

30 days of
YOGA

Day 29

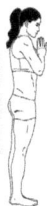

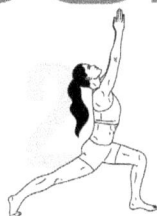

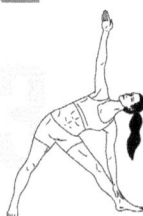

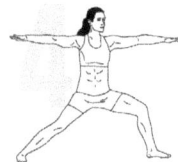

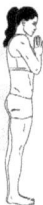

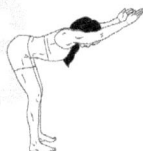

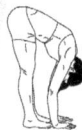

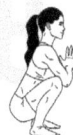

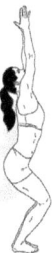

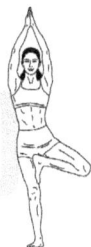

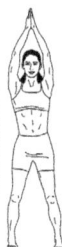

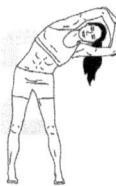

Hold each pose for 20 seconds then move on to the next one.
Repeat the sequence again on the other side.

30. Inner peace

Health benefits of meditation:

- Reduced stress and anxiety
- Improved immune system
- Greater wellbeing
- Improved sleep
- Better health

30 days of
YOGA

Day 30
© darebee.com

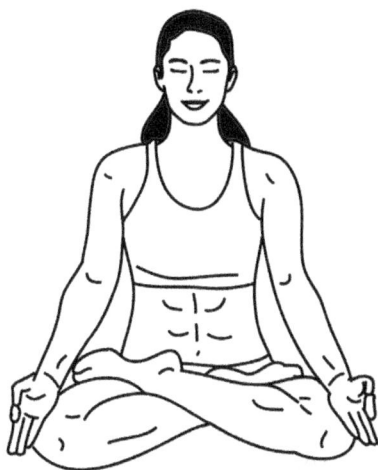

15 minutes
meditation

Angel Workout

When you're looking for a high-burn, aerobically intensive fitness workout that will take you into the sweat zone, Angel delivers. Add EC and you have an extra layer of difficulty to overcome. Make this one a workout to completely conquer.

Extra Credit: 1 minute rest between sets.

ANGEL

DAREBEE WORKOUT © darebee.com

LEVEL I 3 sets **LEVEL II** 5 sets **LEVEL III** 7 sets **REST** up to 2 minutes

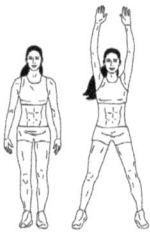

10 jumping jacks

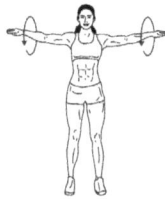

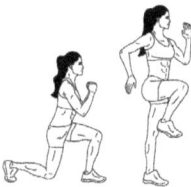

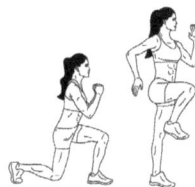

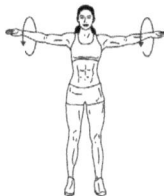

20 raised arm circles

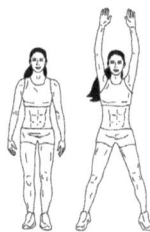

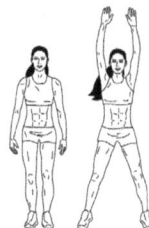

10 jumping jacks

4 lunge step-ups

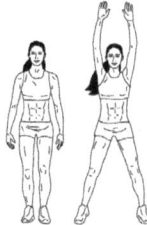

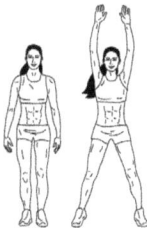

10 jumping jacks

4 lunge step-ups

10 jumping jacks

20 raised arm circles

10 jumping jacks

1 Minute Yoga Challenge

Yoga exercises have amazing effects in the mind and body. You don't need to put in hours and hours to begin to benefit from some of these effects. The 1-minute Yoga, Daily Challenge is a great place to start so you can feel these effects.

1min YOGA

30-Day Challenge

Hold the pose of the day
for 60 seconds in total.

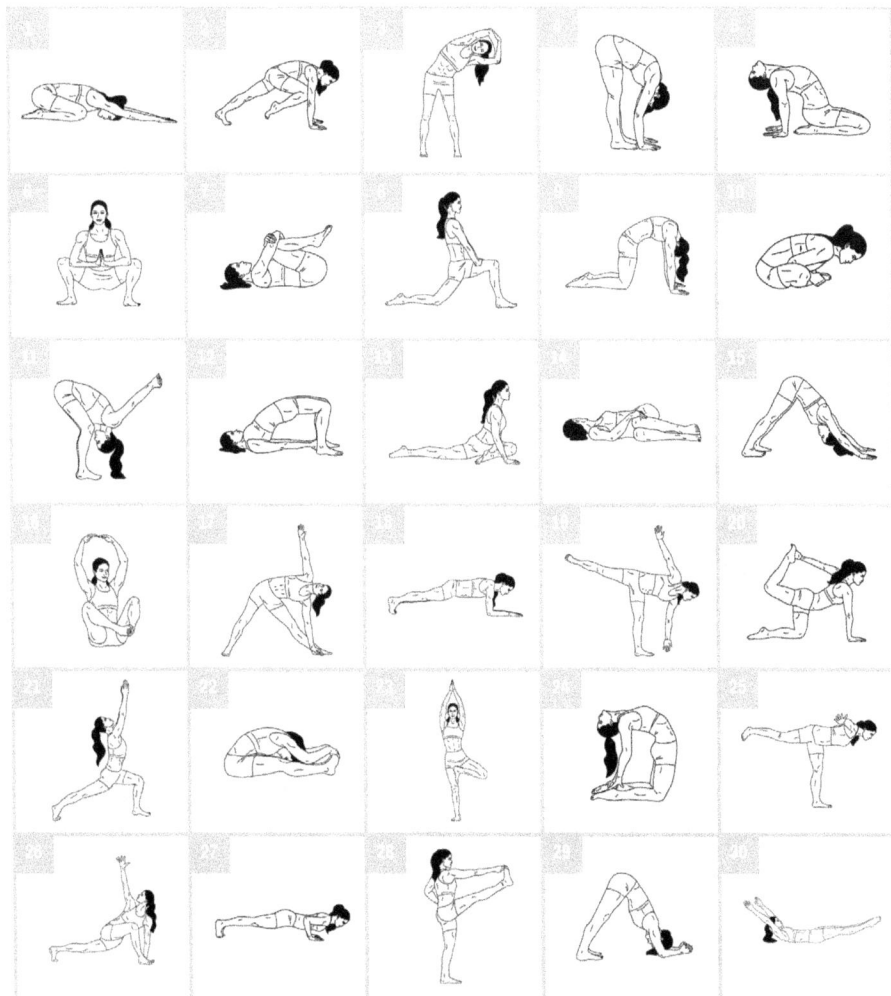

10,000 Crunches Challenge

Muscles trigger their adaptive response and become stronger and more capable in direct response to perceived need. The 10,000 Crunches Challenge creates the perceived need necessary, one day at a time.

You can choose to do all the crunches in one go or separate them into chunks and either do them in installments in one single training session or do them in chunks, throughout the day. The goal is to get to the total number required by the end of the day.

10,000

30-DAY CHALLENGE **CRUNCHES** split total reps into manageable sets © darebee.com

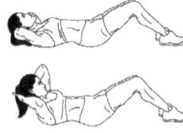

140 crunches	160 crunches	200 crunches	100 crunches	200 crunches
220 crunches	260 crunches	100 crunches	300 crunches	320 crunches
360 crunches	100 crunches	400 crunches	420 crunches	460 crunches
100 crunches	460 crunches	480 crunches	500 crunches	100 crunches
500 crunches	520 crunches	540 crunches	100 crunches	540 crunches
560 crunches	580 crunches	100 crunches	580 crunches	600 crunches

Balance Challenge

A better sense of balance will help you do every physical task better. Because balance is the result of a mind/body loop it will also help you develop better awareness of your body, the way it moves, feels and works and a better grasp of how your brain controls all this.

Instructions: Balance hold time is a total, change legs halfway through e.g., 4 minutes = 2 minutes per leg. Don't put your leg down during in one go side leg raises.

balance

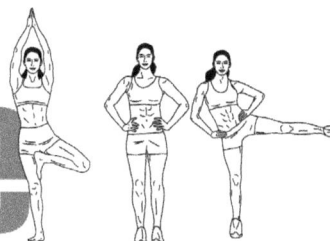

30-DAY CHALLENGE balance hold time is a total, change legs halfway through © darebee.com

3 minutes in one go balance hold	**80** side leg raises throughout the day	**4 minutes** in total balance hold	**80** side leg raises 40/40 in one go	**4 minutes** in one go balance hold
100 side leg raises throughout the day	**5 minutes** in total balance hold	**100** side leg raises 50/50 in one go	**5 minutes** in one go balance hold	**120** side leg raises throughout the day
6 minutes in total balance hold	**120** side leg raises 60/60 in one go	**6 minutes** in one go balance hold	**140** side leg raises throughout the day	**7 minutes** in total balance hold
140 side leg raises 70/70 in one go	**7 minutes** in one go balance hold	**160** side leg raises throughout the day	**8 minutes** in total balance hold	**160** side leg raises 80/80 in one go
8 minutes in one go balance hold	**180** side leg raises throughout the day	**9 minutes** in total balance hold	**180** side leg raises 90/90 in one go	**9 minutes** in one go balance hold
200 side leg raises throughout the day	**10 minutes** in total balance hold	**200** side leg raises 100/100 in one go	**10 minutes** in one go balance hold	**2 min** hold followed up by **200** side leg raises

Get To Bed On Time Challenge

Science tells us that sleep is important for brain health. It is also the time the body uses to repair itself and build muscle. Yet our civilization suffers from a sleep deficit. Life, work and fun conspire to get in the way, creating a 24-hour lifestyle that takes its toll on our physical, mental and psychological health. The Get To Bed Challenge redresses the balance.

Aim to get to bed on time, for a month. Feel the difference that will make to your overall sense of wellbeing.

Get To Bed on time

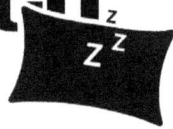

I've got this.	Nice and cosy.	Bed time it is.	I am getting all my Zzz's tonight.	Dear Bed, I love you.
Tomorrow is another day.	Do not disturb	All I need is sleep.	I am going to dream big tonight.	INHALE EXHALE
Keep calm and go to bed.	I deserve more sleep.	I will take over the world. Tomorrow.	Charging time	Sleep solves everything.
My sleep game is strong.	Status: In bed.	I will feel so much better in the morning.	..but first sleep.	3...2...1
I can and I will. SLEEP.	This one is for me.	In bed on time? Check.	The lion sleeps (well) tonight...	Aaand pause.
It's time.	It will all be better tomorrow.	Stronger in the morning.	It makes a difference.	Achievement Unlocked!

Glutes Of Steel Workout

Glutes are the engines that power your body as it walks, sprints, jumps and kicks. The glute is made up of three muscle groups: gluteus maximus, gluteus medius and gluteus minimus. The three muscles originate from the ilium and sacrum and insert on the femur. This makes them part of the connective tissues that keep the upper and lower body functioning as a whole, indivisible unit. Strong glutes make you less prone to fatigue from physical exertion. They significantly contribute to developing explosive power in the lower body and act as one of the conduits that transfer power from the lower body to the upper one. All, in all, strong glutes help you move more confidently and be in greater control of your body. The Glutes of Steel Challenge helps you achieve all this in an incremental, month-long, daily practise.

glutes *of* steel

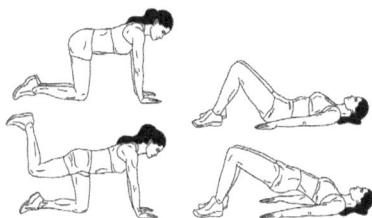

30-Day Challenge
© darebee.com

12 bridges 3 sets in total 30 sec rest between sets	40 leg extensions in total	12 bridges 3 sets in total 30 sec rest between sets	40 leg extensions in total	14 bridges 3 sets in total 30 sec rest between sets
50 leg extensions in total	14 bridges 3 sets in total 30 sec rest between sets	50 leg extensions in total	16 bridges 3 sets in total 30 sec rest between sets	60 leg extensions in total
16 bridges 3 sets in total 30 sec rest between sets	60 leg extensions in total	18 bridges 3 sets in total 30 sec rest between sets	70 leg extensions in total	18 bridges 3 sets in total 30 sec rest between sets
70 leg extensions in total	20 bridges 3 sets in total 30 sec rest between sets	80 leg extensions in total	20 bridges 3 sets in total 30 sec rest between sets	80 leg extensions in total
22 bridges 3 sets in total 30 sec rest between sets	90 leg extensions in total	22 bridges 3 sets in total 30 sec rest between sets	90 leg extensions in total	24 bridges 3 sets in total 30 sec rest between sets
100 leg extensions in total	24 bridges 3 sets in total 30 sec rest between sets	100 leg extensions in totall	26 bridges 3 sets in total 30 sec rest between sets	100 leg extensions in total

No Sugar Challenge

Although our taste buds and our body are highly attuned to the pleasure derived from sugar, today there is sugar in many of our foodstuffs and way too much in our diet. This causes problems with our microbiome, it affects our weight and it impacts on our health. The No Sugar challenge helps you address this balance. Over a month, you help your taste buds reset, you aid in the recovery and resetting of your microbiome flora and discover just how much this small dietary change can affect your weight. You build up a new, healthier you by making small changes, one day at a time. This is a good start.

No Sugar

15-DAY CHALLENGE

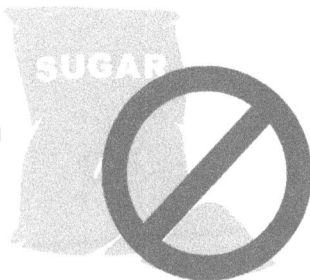

no chocolate,
no cookies,
no soft drinks

© darebee.com

1 I was strong today.	**2** What do I say to chocolate? Not today.	**3** I can always eat it tomorrow.	**4** Nope.	**5** This isn't that difficult. Right? .. Right?
6 Right.	**7** It's been a week. I've got this.	**8** I am stronger today than yesterday.	**9** Every day counts.	**10** They said I can't do it. Watch me.
11 This is nothing. Another day down.	**12** I wasn't about to give up this close to finish. Done.	**13** This isn't even my final form. Done!	**14** One more day. I can do this.	**15** I did it. Woohoo!

Wall-Sit Challenge

Wall Sit is an exercise that pits the power of your quads and the ability of your brain to focus and not give in to fatigue against the gravity of the planet, trying to drag you down.

To succeed you have to fight gravity on a daily basis for incrementally increasing periods of time. The reward for your efforts are noticeably stronger legs and a mind that can focus sufficiently to overcome the limitations of the body.

WALL-SIT

30-DAY CHALLENGE © darebee.com

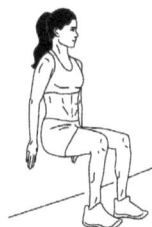

20 seconds wall-sit	**30 seconds** wall-sit	**40 seconds** wall-sit	**20 seconds** wall-sit	**50 seconds** wall-sit
60 seconds wall-sit	**1min 10sec** wall-sit	**20 seconds** wall-sit	**1min 20sec** wall-sit	**1min 30sec** wall-sit
1min 40sec wall-sit	**20 seconds** wall-sit	**1min 50sec** wall-sit	**2 minutes** wall-sit	**2min 10sec** wall-sit
20 seconds wall-sit	**2min 20sec** wall-sit	**2min 30sec** wall-sit	**2min 40sec** wall-sit	**20 seconds** wall-sit
2min 50sec wall-sit	**3 minutes** wall-sit	**3min 10sec** wall-sit	**20 seconds** wall-sit	**3min 20sec** wall-sit
3min 30sec wall-sit	**3min 40sec** wall-sit	**20 seconds** wall-sit	**3min 50sec** wall-sit	**4 minutes** wall-sit

Yoga Abs Challenge

As the difficulty of the challenge increases throughout the 30 days you are guaranteed to feel every second of it. During the final five seconds of each set is when you will be gaining the most. Try to keep it up! It'll be worth it.

Instructions: Add this challenge to your everyday training at the end of your session. It'll make an ideal finisher. After the boat pose hold, slowly transition to knee hug and hold it for the same amount of time. Transition like this 3 times in total (3 sets) to complete the challenge for the day. Don't forget to tighten your core, if you can. If you can't, it's not quite there yet but that's why you are working on it! With consistency and determination you will feel and see your abs in no time. Use the custom timer above to set the time.

Tip: To make the challenge harder change the boat hold to hollow hold. It'll increase the difficulty and subsequently improve the end result.

yoga abs

30-DAY CHALLENGE

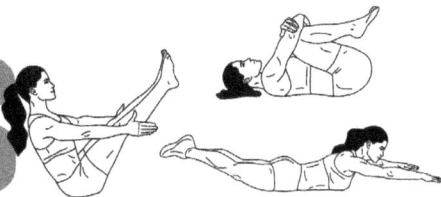

© darebee.com

1	2	3	4	5
20sec boat pose **20sec** knee hug 3 sets	**20sec** superman **20sec** rest 3 sets	**20sec** boat pose **20sec** knee hug 3 sets	**20sec** superman **20sec** rest 3 sets	**25sec** boat pose **25sec** knee hug 3 sets
6	7	8	9	10
25sec superman **25sec** rest 3 sets	**25sec** boat pose **25sec** knee hug 3 sets	**25sec** superman **25sec** rest 3 sets	**30sec** boat pose **30sec** knee hug 3 sets	**30sec** superman **30sec** rest 3 sets
11	12	13	14	15
30sec boat pose **30sec** knee hug 3 sets	**30sec** superman **30sec** rest 3 sets	**35sec** boat pose **35sec** knee hug 3 sets	**35sec** superman **35sec** rest 3 sets	**35sec** boat pose **35sec** knee hug 3 sets
16	17	18	19	20
35sec superman **35sec** rest 3 sets	**40sec** boat pose **40sec** knee hug 3 sets	**40sec** superman **40sec** rest 3 sets	**40sec** boat pose **40sec** knee hug 3 sets	**40sec** superman **40sec** rest 3 sets
21	22	23	24	25
45sec boat pose **45sec** knee hug 3 sets	**45sec** superman **45sec** rest 3 sets	**45sec** boat pose **45sec** knee hug 3 sets	**45sec** superman **45sec** rest 3 sets	**50sec** boat pose **50sec** knee hug 3 sets
26	27	28	29	30
50sec superman **50sec** rest 3 sets	**50sec** boat pose **50sec** knee hug 3 sets	**50sec** superman **50sec** rest 3 sets	**60sec** boat pose **60sec** knee hug 3 sets	**60sec** superman **60sec** rest 3 sets

Amazon Workout

Lower body strength, explosive moves, agility and grace are all part of the Amazon's armory of skills. This is a workout that pushes you from one peak to the other as successive exercises target muscle groups, making different demands on each one. Learn to combine different fitness attributes and seize control of your body.

Amazon

DAREBEE WORKOUT © darebee.com

LEVEL I 3 sets **LEVEL II** 5 sets **LEVEL III** 7 sets **REST** up to 2 minutes

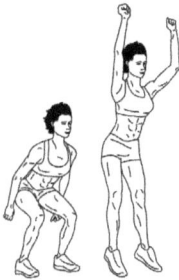

5 jump squats

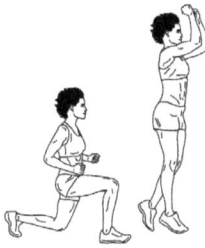

10 jumping lunges

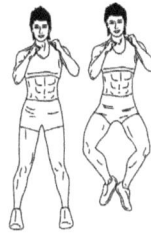

5 hop heel clicks

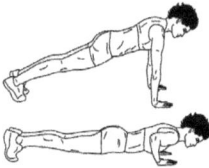

10 push-ups

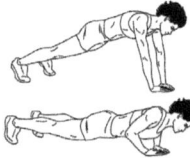

2 close grip push-ups

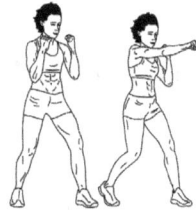

20 punches

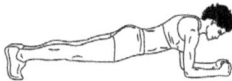

20sec elbow plank

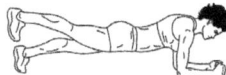

20sec raised leg plank

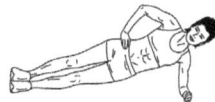

20sec side plank

Atalanta Workout

The Atalanta workout puts your body through its paces testing muscles, tendons, core and abs, coordination, strength, stability and form. Go slow, go full and be deliberate. Focus on how your body moves and your muscles work and try to get as close as possible to perfect form in each execution and yes, that also includes your breathing.

Atalanta

DAREBEE WORKOUT © darebee.com

LEVEL I 3 sets **LEVEL II** 5 sets **LEVEL III** 7 sets **REST** up to 2 minutes

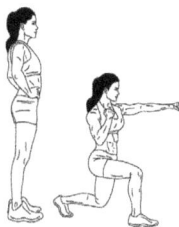

20 lunge punches

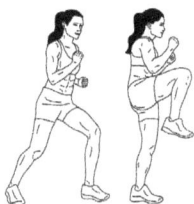

20 knee strikes

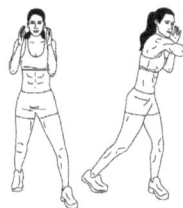

20 elbow strikes

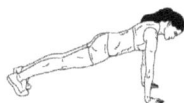
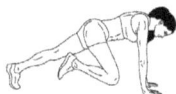

20 slow climbers

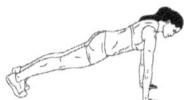
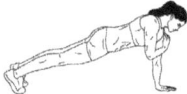

20 shoulder taps

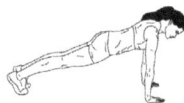
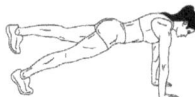

20 plank leg raises

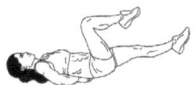
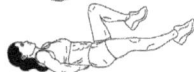

10 bicycle crunches

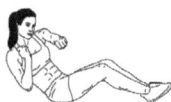
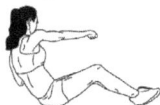

10 sitting punches

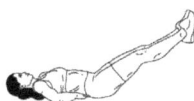
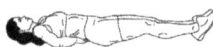

10 leg raises

Swan Workout

Ballet looks deceptively easy but anyone who has tried it knows it is exceptionally difficult requiring great balance, strength, flexibility and coordination, not to mention endurance. Ballet training is great for dancers, obviously, but it is also used by martial artists and boxers who need to move more creatively in very limited space. Try it and get to work muscles of your body you've never used properly, before.

Swan

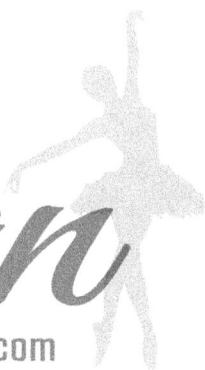

DAREBEE WORKOUT © darebee.com

LEVEL I 3 sets **LEVEL II** 5 sets **LEVEL III** 7 sets **REST** up to 2 minutes

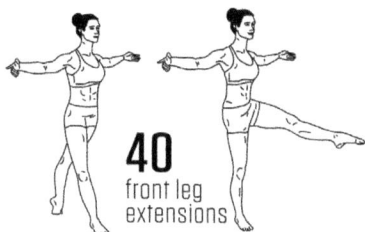

40 front leg extensions

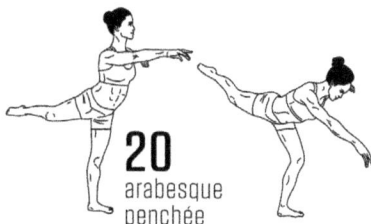

20 arabesque penchée

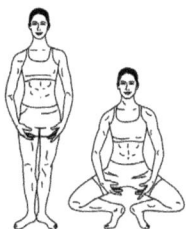

10 grand plié in first position

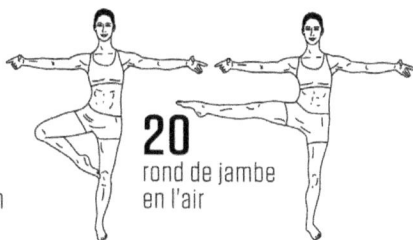

20 rond de jambe en l'air

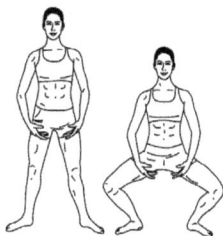

10 grand plié in second position

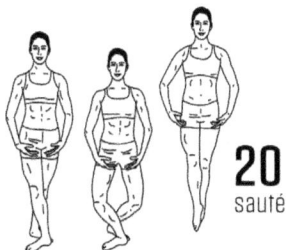

20 sauté

Band It Workout

If you add one willing body and a power stretch band and some time you end up with a whole body band workout that will let you target every major muscle group you need. It requires virtually no space and because the targeting of the muscles is dynamic resistance where they are being asked to work their normal range of movement under an extra load provided by the resistance band. The only problem with the Bandit workout is that it's so hard to resist it should be illegal.

BAND*it*

DAREBEE WORKOUT © darebee.com

LEVEL I 3 sets **LEVEL II** 4 sets **LEVEL III** 5 sets **REST** up to 2 minutes

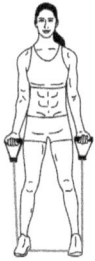

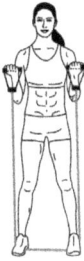

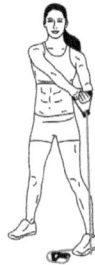

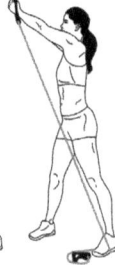

10 bicep curls　　**10** squats　　**10** cross body reach

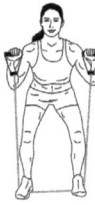

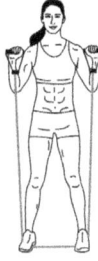

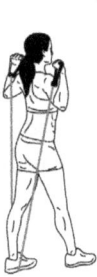

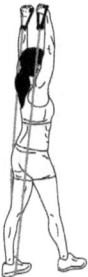

5 shoulder stretch　　**10** tricep extensions　　**5** upright rows

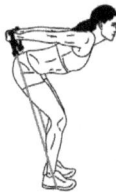

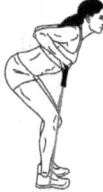

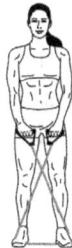

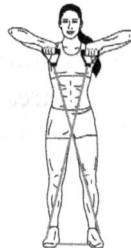

Booty Builder Workout

Glutes are such powerful engines when it comes to athletic performance that it's a wonder we don't do a lot more exercises that focus on building them up. Booty Builder is a workout focused on exactly this area. As a Level II workout it is unlikely to leave you floundering with exhaustion but it won't make you feel like you haven't worked out either, especially if you add EC.

Booty Builder

DAREBEE WORKOUT © darebee.com
2 minutes rest between exercises

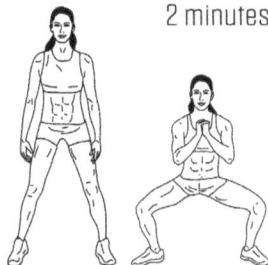

20 wide squats **x 4 sets** in total
20 seconds rest between sets

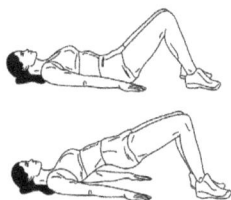

20 bridges **x 4 sets** in total
20 seconds rest between sets

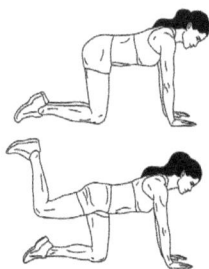

40 leg extensions **x 2 sets** in total
1 set per leg, no rest between sets

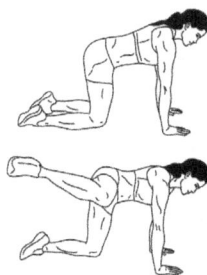

40 side leg extensions **x 2 sets** in total
1 set per leg, no rest between sets

Cellulite Workout

Tighten up muscles, increase tendon control, improve overall circulation, tighten up connective tissue and help get rid of cellulite on legs, glutes and thigh areas as part of an overall fat cell reduction strategy in the body. The Cellulite workout is designed to help you achieve just that while also increasing the control you feel over your body and how you move it. Add EC and it becomes even more challenging.

CELLULITE
WORKOUT

by DAREBEE
© darebee.com

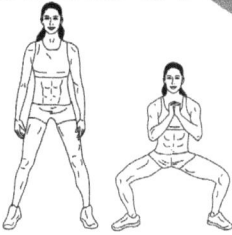

10 wide squats **x 3 sets** in total
30 seconds rest between sets

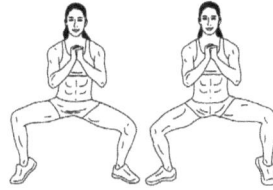

10 squat hold calf raises **x 3 sets** in total
30 seconds rest between sets

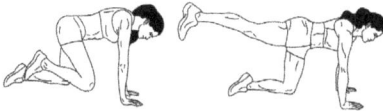

20 back kicks **x 3 sets** in total
30 seconds rest between sets

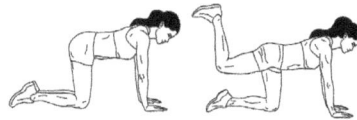

20 leg extensions **x 3 sets** in total
30 seconds rest between sets

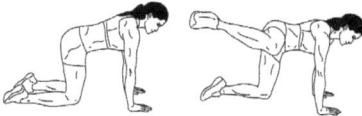

20 side leg extensions **x 3 sets** in total
30 seconds rest between sets

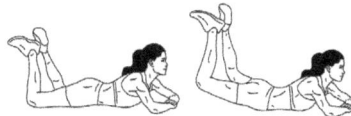

10 glute flex **x 3 sets** in total
30 seconds rest between sets

Chimera Workout

The Chimera workout is a mixed beast of a fitness routine. It uses a complete set of exercise to challenge tendon strength, activate muscles, push the cardiovascular system and make the core stronger. The only thing that'd make it better is your doing the entire routine at level III, twice.

CHIMERA

DAREBEE WORKOUT © darebee.com

LEVEL I 3 sets **LEVEL II** 5 sets **LEVEL III** 7 sets **REST** up to 2 minutes

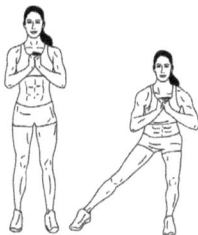

20 side-to-side lunges

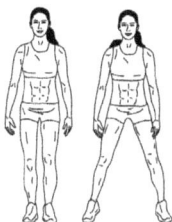

20combos half jack + side leg raise

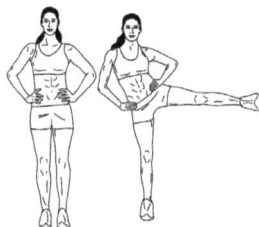

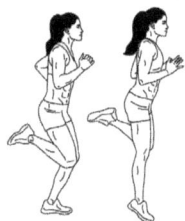

10 butt kicks

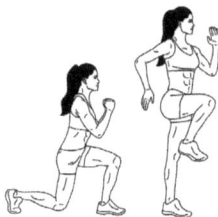

10 lunge step-ups

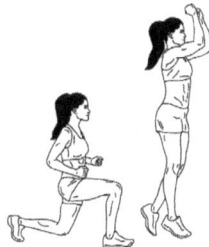

10 jumping lunges

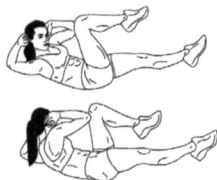

10 knee-to-elbow crunches

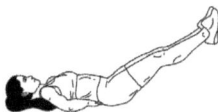

10-count raised leg hold

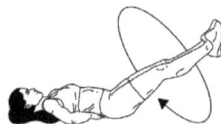

10 raised leg circles

Femme Fatale Workout

Get into character, be a special agent and feel empowered, capable and dangerous with the Femme Fatale workout. Combat moves, groundwork and tendon strengthening exercises will transform your body into one focused, fit, fighting machine. Go for EC and add this workout to your favorites.

FEMME FATALE

DAREBEE
WORKOUT
© darebee.com
LEVEL I 3 sets
LEVEL II 5 sets
LEVEL III 7 sets
2 minutes rest

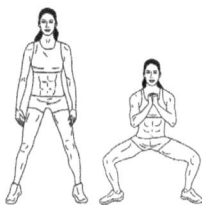

10 goblet squats

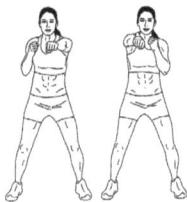

20 punches

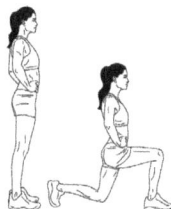

10 lunges

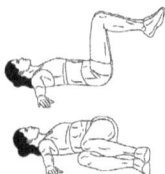

10 half wipers

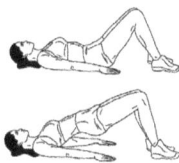

10 bridges

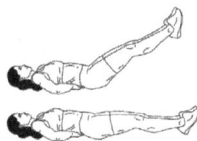

10 leg raises

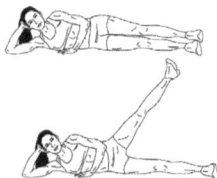

20 side leg raises

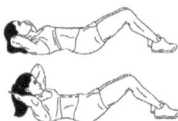

20 crunches

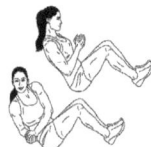

20 sitting twists

Wildfire Workout

Wildfire is a workout designed to make you reach the sweatzone fast and then stay there for as long as you are doing it. It recruits many of the major muscle groups and moves them fast to deliver a targeted, high-burn workout that can only get tougher if you add the EC requirement.

WILDFIRE

DAREBEE CARDIO WORKOUT © darebee.com

LEVEL I 3 sets **LEVEL II** 5 sets **LEVEL III** 7 sets **REST** up to 2 minutes

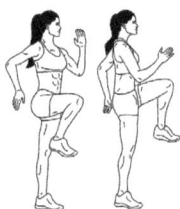
20 march steps

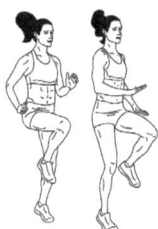
20 high knees

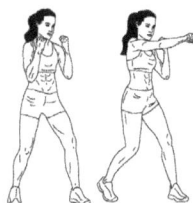
20 punches

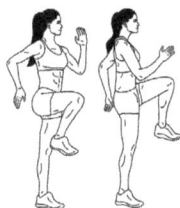
20 march steps

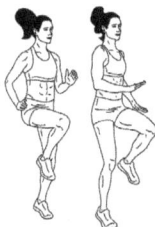
20 high knees

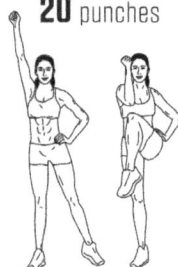
20 knee-to-elbow

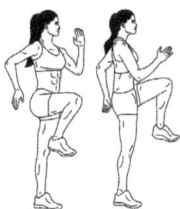
20 march steps

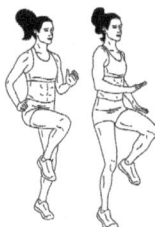
20 high knees

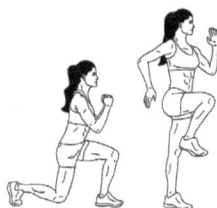
20 lunge step-ups

Wild Child Workout

Wild Child is a fast-moving, pulse-raising, cardiovascular health-improving workout that looks deceptively easy. Raise your knees to waist height during High Knees, make sure your arms are straight as you perform Jumping Jacks and bring your knee to your elbow during Knee-to-Elbow twists and you will see why it looks deceptively easy.

WILD CHILD

DAREBEE WORKOUT © darebee.com
LEVEL I 3 sets **LEVEL II** 5 sets **LEVEL III** 7 sets **REST** up to 2 minutes

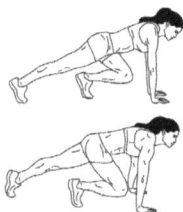

10 climbers

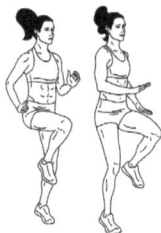

20 high knees

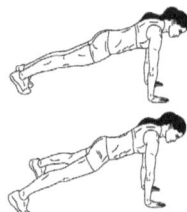

10 plank jacks

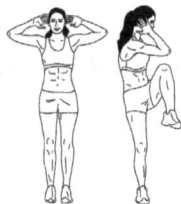

10 knee-to-elbow

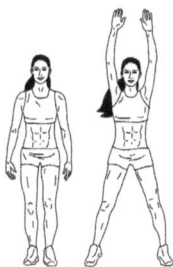

20 jumping jacks

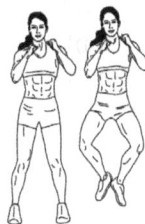

10 hop heel clicks

Valkyrie Workout

Traditionally picked to choose who lived or died in battle Valkyries were warriors in the own right and warriors always need to have the capability to control their bodies and move fast, with grace, under pressure. The Valkyrie workout helps you develop the kind of strength, balance and muscle control that the role requires.

Valkyrie

DAREBEE WORKOUT © darebee.com

LEVEL I 3 sets **LEVEL II** 5 sets **LEVEL III** 7 sets **REST** up to 2 minutes

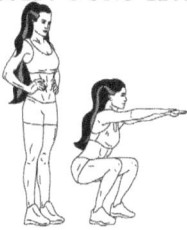

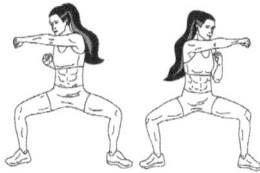

10 squats **10** squat punches **10** squat cross steps

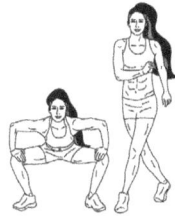

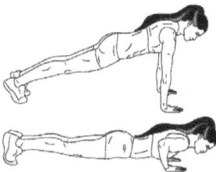

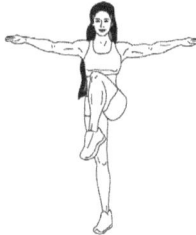

10 push-ups **40sec** balance stand **20** lunge step-ups

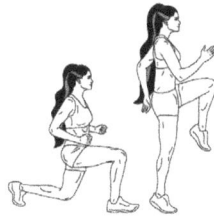

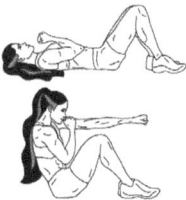

10 sit-up punches **10** crunch kicks **10** side Vs

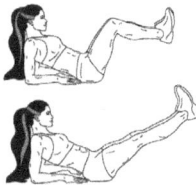

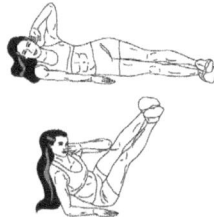

What Doesn't Kill You

You will ask how is it possible for a workout titles What Doesn't Kill You to be only a difficulty level two workout? The answer is to be found only when you reach the seventh set of Level III and have added EC. Really. Try it.

What doesn't Kill you

DAREBEE WORKOUT
© darebee.com
Level I 3 sets
Level II 5 sets
Level III 7 sets
2 minutes rest

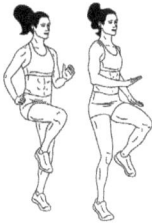

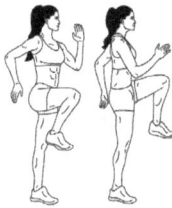

20 high knees   **20** march steps   **20** high knees

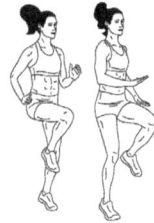

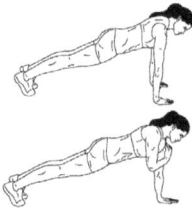

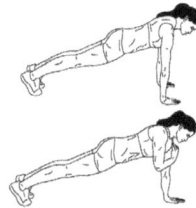

20 shoulder taps   **20** climbers   **20** shoulder taps

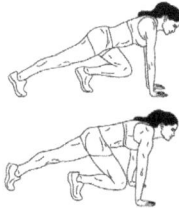

Thank you!

Thank you for purchasing Athena's Playbook, DAREBEE project print edition. DAREBEE is a non-profit global fitness resource dedicated to making fitness accessible for everyone, no matter their circumstances. The project is supported exclusively via user donations and paperback royalties.

After printing costs and bookstore fees every book developed by the DAREBEE project makes $1 and it goes directly into our project maintenance and development fund.

Each sale helps us keep the DAREBEE resource growing, maintain it and keep it up. Thank you for making a difference in its future!

Other books in this series include:

- 100 No-Equipment Workouts Vol 1.
- 100 No-Equipment Workouts Vol 2.
- 100 No-Equipment Workouts Vol 3.
- 100 Office Workouts
- Pocket Workouts: 100 no-equipment workouts
- ABS 100 Workouts: Visual Easy-To-Follow ABS Exercise Routines for All Fitness Levels
- Hero's Journey: 60 Day Fitness Quest: Take part in a journey of self-discovery, changing yourself physically and mentally along the way
- Fighter's Codex: 30-Day At Home Martial Arts Training Program
- 365 Daily Dares: Micro-Fitness For Everyone from Darebee